CARE-FULL

Skills for School Staff to Promote Student Resilience and Prevent Trauma

Textbook

Chelsea Prax, MPH, CPH

AFT | Washington, D.C.

ISBN: 978-8-218-82057-2

First edition

Published by AFT
555 New Jersey Ave. N.W., Washington, DC 20001
aft.org

Cover design by Amy Darling

Printed in the United States of America

Table of Contents

All societal challenges find their way into our schools. Rather than pretending they do not exist, we lean into supporting educators who are helping their students navigate through them. The AFT has created tools and benefits for our members—such as through our student trauma course and our trauma counseling benefit—so they are not alone or isolated as they support their students and our communities. That's what it means to be CARE-FULL: Members turn union resources into welcoming and safe classrooms, campuses and communities where students and families can learn and thrive.

—Randi Weingarten, AFT President

Introduction

In one season of my life, I was trained as an English teacher and worked with high school students. The strategies I learned for supporting English language learners were *good teaching* for all my students—and especially helpful for ELLs.

After working as a teacher, I went on to earn a master's degree and certification in public health. One of my favorite concepts from that training is on universal primary prevention, or the good stuff we can do for everyone, all the time, to promote well-being—without knowing anything about their current health status or future risk profile. The trauma-informed practices we review in this book are akin to those good teaching practices for ELLs and are almost entirely universal primary prevention. In other words, these are best practice for all children, all the time—and they are *especially* helpful for young people grappling with trauma.

AFT is committed to building educators' skills in trauma-informed practice. Research shows that these strategies and initiatives directly promote students' mental health. Additionally, a trauma-informed lens has been linked to improved school safety, staff satisfaction, equity and liberation.

This text is a companion to AFT's graduate-level professional learning course, also titled CARE-FULL.* Here, I endeavor to offer clear, practical synthesis of relevant research, as well as provocative and key ideas that challenge the "center" and the "margins" of our contemporary society. Course participants review and process the information within the book in realistic contexts. They use case studies, discussions, role plays, videos, interactive analysis and more to practice and strengthen the skills discussed in the book.

Professional learning should challenge you to think critically, such as by synthesizing and analyzing disparate materials and ideas. Sometimes this text may make you uncomfortable and that's okay. In the book and the course, in addition to practical approaches and real-world application, I intend to directly confront power, both in the ways that it can be wielded to harm and the ways that it can be transformed for justice. Given the topic, I must also address the negative sides of life, including those for children. I ask you to sit with violence, mortality, oppression and other forms of harm. I ask that you try to get comfortable being uncomfortable, not for the sake of disquiet, but for the transformations that happen when we deliberately examine and even step away from the familiar (MacPhail, 2024).

*A note on the title: I first encountered the term "care-full" in *Care Work: Dreaming Disability Justice* by Leah Lakshmi Piepzna-Samarasinha. Their book is filled with gorgeous, complex musings around disability justice and calls to practice now for the future we want.

Chapters are titled to focus on trauma-informed skills; trauma-informed educators "Stop bullying" and "Support grieving students" and "Reduce the risk of abuse." In each chapter, you'll find:

- **Content notes:** These brief notes are designed to help you decide how and when you might engage with content that may be personally challenging or even triggering. Please ask your facilitators for support to use content notes to structure engagement. For example, "The note says that we'll be covering ____. That's complicated and often stressful for me. Can you help me avoid graphic and vivid content on this topic, please?"
- **A grounding quote:** I share some of the punchy sentences that have helped me coalesce big ideas
- **A synthesis and review of key concepts:** I've attempted to be thorough but not exhaustive. Citations are almost exclusively taken from resources published in the last 10 years. And I lean into robust citation as political practice
- **At least one reflection question** to guide continued thoughtful engagement
- **A recommended resource:** I approached this section with the question, "If I could only suggest one item for continued learning, which would it be?" Use the chapter's citations to develop a lengthier syllabus as you see fit

I hope you use each chapter in whichever order best suits you to deepen your commitment and capacities for children's well-being. Thank you for meeting me here.

—Chelsea Prax

Psychological safety

> *"This is not a place for healing, though healing may happen here."*
> —Kazu Haga (Healing Resistance, 2020)

Learning about, talking about and making meaning of stressful, harmful and traumatic experiences can be upsetting. The goal of this text is not to upset anyone, yet readers (and participants in the paired AFT professional learning course) may experience unpleasant and even triggering moments. To promote psychological safety for readers, course participants and facilitators, CARE-FULL materials and facilitators endeavor to:

- Limit graphic, vivid and detailed material about specific types or instances of trauma.
- Use content notes to invite and inform your consent to engage.
- Separate takeaway content from engagement activities.
- Practice reasonable boundaries and promote access to complementary union benefits.

CARE-FULL materials and facilitators **limit graphic, vivid and detailed material.**

This text is designed to share information and to help readers understand skills to promote children's health and well-being. The research reviewed here focuses on ways of thinking and acting that help people—who may or may not have an illness—"tilt toward wellness," no matter their starting point. This text does not offer strategies to manage, treat or cure illness.

Relatedly, you may encounter realistic examples and poignant profiles, including references to specific mental health challenges, such as anxiety, depression or post-traumatic stress disorder. Use these to envision real-world opportunities to consider how you might shift practice. We do not have therapeutic keys to specific diagnoses. Rather, the strategies elevated here are *universal, tier 1 approaches*—good for all adults in school to use with all students all the time.

CARE-FULL materials and facilitators **use content notes.**

We invite your consent to engage in challenging material by acknowledging potentially upsetting and triggering subject matter. Content notes tell you in advance about topics we'll cover that may distress you. They are not *clinical* or *therapeutic*; they will not help you or students heal. They are not designed to make you feel better. They do not stop you from having strong reactions. They will not necessarily make it easier to engage with a topic. They are an effort to alert you to moments when you may need to prioritize taking care of yourself, such as by pacing differently or identifying a buddy who can help you debrief what you review. Please use content notes to help you proactively decide how and when you will engage in subjects that may be especially challenging.

CARE-FULL materials and facilitators **separate takeaway content from engagement activities.**

Based on robust feedback from previous participants in the AFT professional learning on "Student Trauma," we have endeavored to make substantive content available in this textbook. Please periodically return to the text and ethically share!

- Review and share textbook content, including the "recommended resource" that closes each chapter.
- Build a syllabus for deeper engagement by reviewing citations.
- Limit storytelling to *your* course experiences; observe reasonable boundaries and confidentiality for other participants.

Much like completing a university course does not make you a professor, engaging with CARE-FULL content and activities does not make you an AFT facilitator. **Even well-intentioned sharing of course materials could re-traumatize and cause harm** (Vickers, 2019; Fisher, 1999). Readers should not capture, reproduce, adapt, sell or share course materials with the intent to disseminate as training or professional development resources.

CARE-FULL materials and facilitators **practice reasonable boundaries.**

As you engage with this text, you may have deep personal realizations. This book and the course facilitators do not offer support to actively process personal trauma or specific instances of student trauma. Course facilitators do not coordinate clinical care. They are prepared to support you with skills they have and to help streamline access to relevant union benefits. Check out an overview of the AFT Trauma Counseling Benefit on the next page.

Note: If you are interested in accessing the course facilitation manual, leading activities, assisting with course revision or another form of deep engagement, request your union leadership's support to join an AFT training of facilitators event. National facilitators undertake additional preparation and receive ongoing coaching, as well as content resources that help them develop expertise and avoid the potential harm of misusing course materials.

AFT Trauma Counseling Benefit

Frequently asked questions

Q: What is trauma counseling?

A: Trauma counseling is an innovative form of mental health care that provides confidential therapy at any time in the one-year aftermath of a traumatic incident. It matches you with a therapist and uses the latest communication technologies—phone, video, text and even AI (artificial intelligence)—to provide help when you need it.

Q: Who is eligible?

A: All AFT members who are either actively employed or on a leave of absence and who have experienced a covered traumatic incident are eligible to receive this benefit. Retired members and agency fee payers are not eligible for this coverage.

Q: What is covered and when?

A: You are covered 24 hours a day, 365 days a year, if your incident involves any of the following: domestic violence, aggravated assault, sexual assault, mass shooting or terrorism, or you are infected, injured or traumatized by a disease during a FEMA-declared major disaster. Coverage also includes incidents in your place of work if you are traumatized by contracting an infectious disease, witnessing a violent incident, bullying, harassment, threats or secondary traumas.

Q: What is considered a major disaster?

A: There are two types of disaster declarations made by the federal government: emergency declarations and major disaster declarations. A major disaster is any natural catastrophe, including any hurricane, tornado, storm, high water, wind-driven water, tidal wave, tsunami, earthquake, volcanic eruption, landslide, mudslide, snowstorm or drought, or, regardless of cause, any fire, flood or explosion in any part of the United States, that causes damage, ecological disruption, loss of human life and deterioration of health and health services on a large scale.

Q: Didn't I already have this benefit?

A: This is an additional and unique benefit beyond any provided by your insurance, your employer, an employee assistance program or workers' compensation.

Q: What does this cost?

A: There is no cost to you; it is an AFT-paid benefit for eligible members.

Q: Does the traumatic incident have to occur at work to be eligible to receive the benefit?

A: No. Your coverage is much broader than your employment. Some incidents are specific to the workplace, while others are broader.

Q: How do I sign up? How can I trust that this service is confidential?

A: You do not have to sign up for the service until you need it. Members will gain access to the program through the AFT Member Benefits portal: **aft.org/members-only**. This requires registration with a member ID; after that, you will work directly with the provider. If you need your AFT Member ID, complete this form and we'll send you a registration link: **leadernet.aft.org/webform/aft-members-only-discounts**

Your employer will not be notified that you have sought or received this service. Additionally, your information is fully protected under HIPAA regulations.

Q: Why am I required to submit a claim to receive benefits?

A: Trauma counseling is provided through insurance and submitting a claim is the process to request benefits—like requesting healthcare benefits through your health insurance company.

Q: Is this different from an employee assistance program?

A: Yes, the counselors in this program have all received specialized training in post-traumatic care. The benefit offers up to 21 hours of therapy, personally customized to stretch across three months in short and long sessions, and staged to include a diagnosis, a midway update and a final summarizing session.

Q: What if I don't have access to a computer?

A: Please call the program's toll-free number, 855-631-1421, to speak with an authorized representative about different ways to access this form of therapy.

Q: If I use trauma counseling, can I also receive benefits from workers' compensation, my employer and/or counseling through my insurance?

A: Yes, this trauma benefit is in addition to those benefits.

Q: When is this benefit not available?

A: Coverage ends if you are no longer an AFT member actively employed or on a leave of absence.

Q: Do I need to enroll?

A: Working AFT members are automatically enrolled.

Q: Is there a waiting period?

A: No. Once you successfully register at the AFT member portal, you are immediately eligible to receive this benefit.

Q: How do I find a therapist who is covered by this trauma counseling benefit?

A: You don't have to find a therapist. The trauma counseling program will connect you. It has identified high-performing therapists across the United States. Each is licensed, has earned a master's or higher degree, is trained in post-traumatic incident mental health care and has undergone an extensive background check. If you are currently working with a therapist or have a preferred therapist, you may use this benefit to compensate them directly.

Q: What if I don't have time to see a counselor?

A: Because this counseling is facilitated by today's technology, you have great flexibility in setting up your sessions, which can occur 24/7 from anywhere. Of course, sessions must be scheduled at times agreeable to both parties.

Q: What if I don't seek trauma counseling right after an incident?

A: Trauma counseling can be provided within one year from the date of a covered incident. Counseling must begin within one year following an incident.

Q: Do I have to be an AFT member to get access to this program?

A: Yes. This program is exclusively for AFT members who are actively employed or on leave.

Q: How do I file a claim?

A: Claims can be filed directly on the trauma counseling page reachable via the link at aft.org/members-only. Under plan resources, members will find a Submit a Claim tab. This will enable members to provide more information, along with any documentation needed for the claim.

Q: Where can I find more information about the paid trauma coverage benefit?

A: You can learn more at the Trauma Coverage website, accessible through the portal at **aft.org/members-only** or call Trauma Coverage toll-free at 855-631-1421.

Testimonials

Since 2014, AFT has coordinated professional learning on trauma-informed practices for thousands of educators across the United States. The following testimonials are from participant course evaluations submitted between 2020 and 2024.

"I thoroughly enjoyed the training, the information and resources and having them available after the training is a plus. Thank you for all of the hard work that went into the planning of such a thorough training."

"I was really impressed with this course. The amount of information y'all squeezed into such a short few weeks is admirable. There was no filler; it was all useful research and concrete teaching strategies, and I appreciate not just your hard knowledge and efficient delivery, but the fact that you clearly value your own and my time. I wish all teachers had to take this course! I will do my best to spread what I have learned here. I genuinely look forward to future AFT eLearning opportunities. Thank y'all!"

"I think overall this was the most powerful PD on Trauma informed [sic] strategies I have ever taken."

"Since we shut down our school last March, one of the things required by our district was to log professional development. So after watching hours and hours of TED talks and reading hundreds of hours of studies and strategies, I was of the mindset of "oh here we go again" ... (sorry). To my pleasant surprise I am still reading and reviewing so I can increase what I share with others. It is a truly promising program and I will use it all the time as we move forward through the new frontier of life after the pandemic!"

"I truly enjoyed this course. All three facilitators were affable, welcoming and knowledgeable. I appreciated every bit of information they were able to teach us. If I have any critique, it's that I almost wish this course were longer—maybe an extra week's worth of sessions dedicated to reviewing materials."

"This course provided me with a lot of new mindsets and resources to further my own trauma-informed education and practices. I was able to apply new things in my classroom right away with positive results 100 percent of the time. This course built my confidence in multiple areas and was everything I could have hoped for."

Becoming trauma-informed

Confident, thriving educators acting in strategic and liberatory collaboration are essential to trauma-informed schooling. The first few chapters of this book focus on what it looks like and what it takes for educators to thrive through iterative changes and challenges—both individual and institutional—toward shared visions for healing and justice. Chapters include "Elevate educator wellness," "Strengthen worker relationships for change," "Practice grounding" and "Exercise healthy relational boundaries."

> *"What would it mean to not only say, You hurt me, to not only say I see you, too, have been hurt, but to say: I see that my thriving happens alongside yours? What would it mean to move together, as critical theorist and literary scholar Chad Inante calls us to do, not only in coalition but in collusion?"*
>
> —Eve Ewing (Original Sins: The Miseducation of Black and Native Children and the Construction of American Racism, 2025)

Most educators understand intimately that students' mental health poses incredible challenges and opportunities at school. Mental health is one of educators' top priorities for work on children's well-being (Prax, 2015). Trauma-informed educators go further than naming the problem by learning and practicing key skills to positively promote children's mental health and overall growth:

- **Understand** the ways unaddressed stress and adversity undermine mental health.
- **Prevent** further traumatization by proactively introducing and sustaining protective factors so students learn to navigate issues and grow, rather than shut down.
- **Effectively support** students experiencing unpleasant feelings and human responses to distress.
- **Identify** students who may benefit from more intensive supports.
- **Coordinate** warm and safe learning environments for all students.

- **Balance powerful bonding with ethical boundaries**, so relationships are sustainable, reciprocal and ultimately effective in shifting toward well-being.

Being trauma-informed demands considerable reflection on your worldview, practices and impacts (not just intentions). As you move through the book, you will encounter a variety of skills, ideas and calls to action. Some parts may seem intimate, cozy and familiar; others may seem particularly challenging, new or innovative. Relatedly, some components of being trauma-informed may feel difficult, as if your work requires more complexity or more steps as you plan, deliver, assess and engage students and families. With practice and time, these skills become habits and these shifts become standards.

We begin this book with studious attention to self-actualized educators as one of the most important "ingredients" in trauma-informed schooling. The health, self-efficacy and collaborative capacity of the workforce determines success with all that must follow.

1 Elevate educator wellness

CONTENT NOTE. This chapter includes ideas related to coronavirus pandemic, gun violence, mental illness, physical violence and workplace violence.

"'When people and societies enter into a state of shock, they lose their identities and their footing,' [John Berger] observed. 'Hence, calm is a form of resistance.' Calm is not a replacement for righteous rage or fury at injustice—both of which are powerful drivers for necessary change. But calm is the precondition for focus, for the capacity to prioritize. If shock induced a loss of identity, then calm is the condition under which we return to ourselves."

—Naomi Klein (Doppelganger: A Trip into the Mirror World, 2024)

Workers in different sectors face occupational health hazards unique to their worksites and sector dynamics. Addressing educators' workplace well-being directly influences schools' capacity to implement trauma-informed practices (Jennings, 2015). This chapter focuses on threats to educators' well-being as well as some of the ways that self-care can be protective.

Occupational hazards in education

Educators report more significant stress and worse health than other workers. Nearly 1 in five (18 percent) educators characterized their health as fair or poor on an AFT survey (Educator Quality of Worklife: Executive Summary, 2015). The union also found that educators are nearly twice as likely as other workers to report "not good" mental health in the last 30 days (AFT, 2015). Compared to other U.S. workers, educators are significantly more likely to have been diagnosed with hypertension and blood sugar issues (AFT, 2015; AFT, 2017). Several factors complicate educators' occupational health, including:

- Widespread worries about workplace mass shooting—a concern for 46 percent of educators (Hart Research, 2022)

- Attacks by students and increased aggression from students, parents, colleagues and administrators during crisis events (McMahon, et al., 2022). About 6 percent of educators overall experience such aggression, with elementary educators facing four times the burden [9.3 percent] of secondary educators [2.3 percent] (Irwin, Wang, Cui, Zhang, & Thompson, 2021)
- More job-related stress and symptoms of depression than other workers (Steiner & Woo, 2021; Steiner, et al., 2022)
- Racism and systemic targeting among educators in oppressed groups (Steiner, et al., 2022; Blaustein & Kinniburgh, 2019).

Assess workplace well-being

The Professional Quality of Life (ProQOL) instrument can assist educators to quickly assess and understand workplace well-being. It can also help educators identify when coping mechanisms are overwhelmed: when they are more likely to need support, new strategies or a break from stressors. ProQOL is a free, 30-item self-report measure of the positive and negative aspects of caring. It includes two components:

- 10 questions measure compassion satisfaction, or the positive aspects of working as a helper.
- 20 total questions measure compassion fatigue, or the negative aspects of working as a helper. These questions are split into two subscales:
  - » 10 questions on burnout measure workers' feelings of inefficacy and overwhelm.
  - » 10 questions on secondary trauma examine workers' trauma responses related to supporting someone who directly experienced a traumatic event or exposure.

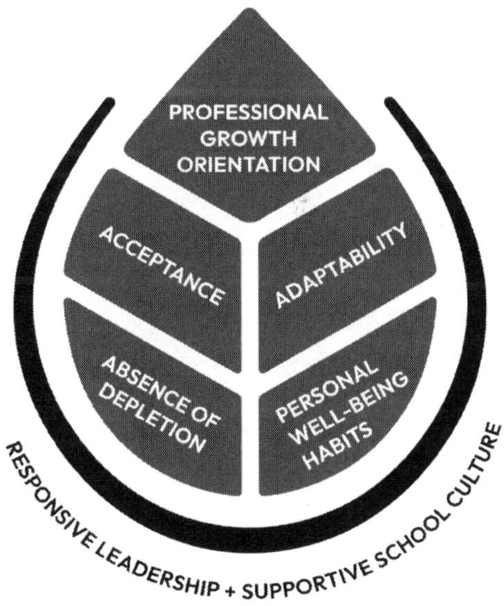

Six Predictive Factors of Well-Being (AFT and Educators Thriving, 2023).

ProQOL is widely used, thoroughly validated, easy to use and score, good for use among individuals or in groups and can be given in a variety of formats. It is not a medical test, psychological test or diagnostic tool. Think of it as a screening for stress-related health problems. The results can help individuals plan where to put energy for increased resilience; results can help organizations strategize; and results can inform discussions about support (Stamm, Higson-Smith, Hudnall, Piland, & Hudnall Stamm, 2012).

The ProQOL instrument has been widely used in research with healthcare workers. However, a few studies focus on the education sector. Educators tend to have high compassion satisfaction and a positive attitude toward their work environment. However, significant proportions of educators also tend to have high levels of compassion fatigue (Darawsheh, Asha, AbuSaif, Alhejoj, & Khasawneh, 2023). Other researchers assert that moderate compassion fatigue is widespread and "needs urgent attention" (Yu, et al., 2022).

In the education sector, risks are not equitably distributed (Ollison, 2019). Women working in education experience more compassion fatigue than men. Compassion fatigue and burnout are more acute in new educators than in veterans. Furthermore, educators with decades of experience tend to report higher compassion satisfaction. Teachers working with marginalized communities—including students living in high-poverty and those facing systemic racism—experience less compassion satisfaction and more compassion fatigue than their counterparts in schools with more mainstream demographics.

Clarify threats

Educators face elevated risk of secondary traumatic stress (STS) and up to 75 percent report STS symptoms (Lawson, Caringi, Gottfried, Bride, & Hydon, 2019). Specialized instructional support personnel (SISP)—such as school counselors, nurses, social workers and psychologists—may be at even higher risk for STS than other educators, as they face repeated exposure to traumatic events through both personal experience and professional care encounters (Lawson, Caringi, Gottfried, Bride, & Hydon, 2019). Furthermore, educators may carry significant and sometimes unaddressed or unmanaged, childhood trauma of their own, compounding the challenge of effectively addressing student trauma (Blaustein & Kinniburgh, 2019).

Sometimes these challenges are lumped into the term "compassion fatigue." It's important to critically reflect on this term and its associations. The ability to be patient, open and present, to form positive and supportive relationships in nurturing professions makes workers in those fields more likely to learn about and be invited to address trauma. More exposure to violence, including through empathic engagement with others' experiences, increases the risk for secondary, or vicarious, trauma. In other words, *compassion* does not put educators at risk. Educators are not "fatigued" by efforts to care or to exist in beloved community. Rather, educators are exhausted by myriad forms of violence that affront human dignity and make it harder to show and experience care. They are fatigued by the need to deeply understand and consistently confront depravity (Mayte, 2023; Trey, 2024).

Despite elevated risks, estimates of trauma among educators—as measured by scores on the Adverse Childhood Experiences questionnaire—are not significantly different from the general adult population (Sweeney & Caringi, 2020; Merrick, Ford, Ports, & Guinn, 2018). These data suggest that educators may be particularly effective at coping with workplace stress, compared to workers in other sectors.

Coping routines

Like tooth brushing and handwashing, regular health promotion practices, such as meditation, drinking sufficient water, eating a nutritious diet, physical activity, sleep routines and wellness visits, are effective for *coping* with stress and trauma (Scotland-Coogan & Davis, 2016; Jennings, 2015). Since they don't necessarily "feel good" or impactful the moment we do them, these strategies are easy to abandon in favor of comfort and avoidance strategies that quickly satisfy the brain's pleasure center.

Alcohol and drug use, shopping sprees, comfort food binges, emotional repression and entertainment are often called "self-care." These help us feel good for a moment or distract from feeling not-so-good ... *and* they can be overused. Taken to extremes, comfort-focused and avoidant strategies thwart good health. People whose "toolkit" for stress coping is primarily about comfort (or avoidance) tend to have higher stress levels and tend to maintain higher stress levels (Bistricky, et al., 2019; Schibalski, et al., 2017).

Reflections

- In your own words, list three hazards to educators' health.
- How do you think educators can balance the need for self-care while also maintaining a high level of care for their students?

Recommended resource

"Beyond Burnout: A Roadmap to Improve Educator Well-Being" by AFT and Educators Thriving, **aft.org/sites/default/files/media/documents/2023/Beyond_Burnout_A_Roadmap_to_Improve_Educator_Wellbeing.pdf**

2 Strengthen worker relationships for change

CONTENT NOTE. This chapter includes ideas related to coronavirus pandemic and workplace violence.

> *"You can't deep-breathe your way out of a pandemic; you cannot stretch your way out of terrible class sizes; you cannot "individual behavior" your way out of structural problems. Those are effective coping measures, but they don't change the problem."*
>
> —Chelsea Prax (Will, 2021)

Educators' well-being isn't just about individual routines, like meditation or exercise; it's also about collective care. This means educators and staff working together to support each other, tackle systemic barriers and create positive change. Schools can build cultures of care by offering professional development, fostering peer support and advocating for changes that promote justice for both educators and students.

Assess your work environment

Coping with challenges at work is not the same as *solving* problems or *addressing* root causes. Many schools admonish educators to practice self-care and achieve their own well-being—to cope. Yet schools often fail to implement universal programming or make policy changes to address staff wellness (Institute of Educational Sciences, 2022). Federal data collected during the coronavirus pandemic suggest that:

- 67 percent of schools made no changes to the academic school year
- Nearly 1 in 3 schools report no social-emotional learning program
- 19 percent of schools offer no benefits related to educators' mental health
- Just 9 percent of schools regularly assess educators' well-being

Educators have strong wellness when they experience being valued and respected as leaders; are deeply engaged in their work; find meaning and purpose in their work; feel successful; have their personal, non-work needs met; manage their emotions and well-being; and experience a positive, supportive work environment (Proeschold-Bell, et al., 2021; AFT and Educators Thriving,

2023). Policies that increase educators' time directly engaging students are also linked to improved positive affect (Jones, Camburn, Kelcey, & Quintero, 2021; DeStigter, 2018).

Systemic > individual change

Educators have long been burdened by rhetoric about "natural" inclinations to care for children and the labor of education as a "calling." These narratives contribute to high demands for educators to offer emotional and intellectual support. They also logically lead many to blame educators for children's imperfect outcomes: "If they demand better conditions for themselves, they're called selfish, even as their demands are often ones that would improve their students' lives as well. Yet teachers have a long history of militant organizing, of challenging the boundaries placed around them by politicians and administrators, and of bringing their communities along with them" (Jaffe, 2021).

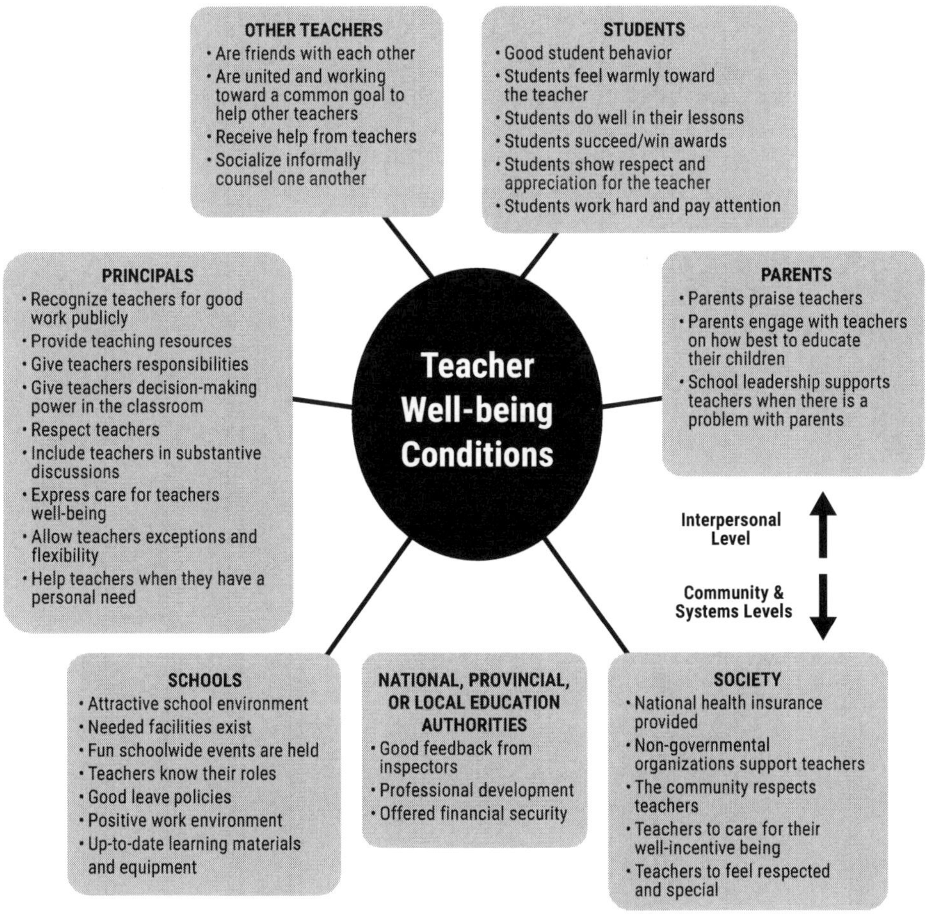

Teacher well-being conditions present in teacher and principal interview data in three contexts (Proeschold-Bell, et al., 2021).

To challenge these outcomes and build on resistance among urban school personnel that started in the nineteenth century, the AFT was founded in 1916 in Chicago. Members wanted to elevate their voices in decision-making alongside that of stakeholders like superintendents and ultimately, achieve democracy in schools (AFTHQ, 2021). In the words of Margaret Haley, a Chicago Teachers Federation (known today as the Chicago Teachers Union) pioneer, "The ideal of democracy, the ideal of the educators, [...] places humanity above all machines, and demands that all activity shall be the expression of life" (Jaffe, 2021).

Shared power in decision-making—such as through labor-management collaboration—is also powerfully linked to educator well-being and retention (Steiner, et al., 2022; AFT and Educators Thriving, 2023). Educators working together can more effectively develop and implement solutions to address staffing and working conditions (McCarthy & Rubinstein, 2018). Moreover, if labor-management collaboration is not possible or successful, working with the union can also help to achieve shared power in decision-making. For example, educators and their unions have teamed up with families to improve quality of life with wins such as desegregated schools, new play spaces and more diverse workforces (Jaffe, 2021; Action Center on Race and the Economy, 2025).

Reflections

Name one person—a colleague, administrator, union representative or student caregiver—with whom you could initiate, strengthen or leverage a relationship toward systemic change for educators' workplace wellness.

Recommended resource

"Restoring Teacher and Principal Well-Being Is an Essential Step for Rebuilding Schools" by Steiner, et al., **rand.org/content/dam/rand/pubs/research_reports/RRA1100/RRA1108-4/RAND_RRA1108-4.pdf**

3 Practice grounding

CONTENT NOTE. This chapter includes ideas related to mental illness and physical illness.

> *"When you take time to savor the good, you simply need less of it."*
>
> —Stephanie Foo (What My Bones Know: A Memoir of Healing from Complex Trauma, 2022)

Stress reduction practices in schools are linked to improved student focus, reduced anxiety symptoms and improved cognitive skills (Dunning, et al., 2022; Pascoe, Thompson, Jenkins, & Ski, 2017). School-based mindfulness programs are also linked to short-term improvements in educator burnout and school climate (Kuyken, et al., 2022). Relaxation techniques may assist in managing over-reactive stress responses, a common traumatic effect (Scotland-Coogan & Davis, 2016).

Before reviewing promising research and practices, we want to encourage critical engagement with school-based stress reduction. While research and news media coverage are nearly unanimously positive, meditation and mindfulness are not a panacea and the evidence is not consistently generated in high-quality studies to corroborate amazing claims. While nothing suggests that meditation is harmful, its effects are comparable to an antidepressant pill without side effects (Jazaieri, 2017). Meditation, mindfulness, coping strategies, resilience and social-emotional learning are absolutely part of supporting students. They must complement—not replace—a commitment to achieving equity and eliminating, wherever possible, the violence and injustice that challenge student development (Venet, 2021).

Mindful meditation

Meditation and mindfulness are overlapping categories with many different components that can be combined for practical application to call gentle, nonjudgmental attention to the mind-body interaction, including (Pascoe, Thompson, Jenkins, & Ski, 2017):

- **Postures:** Seated, laying down, walking
- **Mental practice/content focus:** Guided attention to thoughts (or spaces between thoughts), feelings, bodily sensations, visualizations and/or

external stimuli; mental or silent repetition of a word, phrase, feeling or concept

- **Physical practice:** Structured breathing and/or thought exercises; eyes open or closed; chanting; repetitive finger movement; stretching
- **Environment:** Music, voice or audio cues; alternately, mindfulness can be practiced in silence
- **Duration:** At least 3 minutes

Emotional freedom technique tapping

Also called *EFT tapping*, emotional freedom technique tapping was first developed to help people with anxiety. The practice is linked to significant positive benefits in the short- and long-term, including declines in anxiety, blood pressure, cortisol (a key stress hormone), depression, PTSD and pain, as well as increases in happiness and mental well-being (Bach, et al., 2019). Subsequent research has shown it to be helpful for a wide variety of psychological symptoms, primarily because it helps to quickly reduce stress.

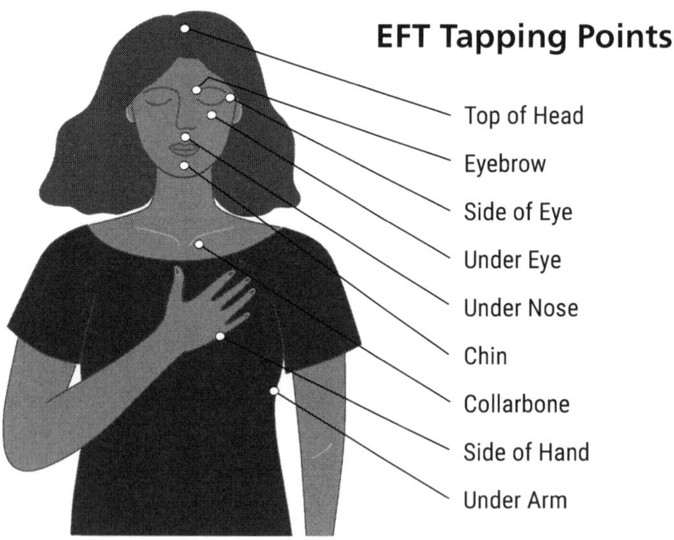

EFT tapping relies on a series of quick and gentle taps on nine acupressure points.

While specific acupressure points are essential to have therapeutic effect, research does not support the use of any specific statements. "Rounds," or cycling through the acupressure points multiple times with a variety of statements, may make EFT tapping more effective (Rogers & Sears, 2015; Church, Stapleton, Yang, & Gallo, 2018).

Physical activity

Rhythmic physical activity helps regulate the body and activity that switches from side-to-side may be particularly calming (Perry, 2020). Educators can support students by consistently and repeatedly using activities like songs and music-based exercises, circle games, drumming, short-bursts of exercise, mindful breathing, visualizations, yoga or tai-chi adaptations, as well as drumming (Brunzell, Waters, & Stokes, 2015).

Cultivating positivity

The broaden-and-build theory posits that positive emotions expand the thought-action repertoire. More specifically:

- **Joy** sparks the urge to play.
- **Interest** sparks the urge to explore.
- **Contentment** sparks the urge to savor and integrate.
- **Love** sparks a recurring cycle of each of these urges within safe, close relationships.

In students, positive emotions build social resources, such as novel and creative actions, ideas and relational bonds, which in turn build an individual's personal resources. Importantly, increased physical, intellectual, social and psychological resources function as reserves that can be accessed later to improve the odds of successful coping (Frederickson, 2004; Brunzell, Waters, & Stokes, 2015). Cultivating positivity also helps educators practice unconditional positive regard and boost student healing (Brunzell, Waters, & Stokes, 2015; Venet, 2021).

Progressive muscle relaxation

After two months of regularly practicing progressive muscle relaxation (once a week for eight weeks), nurses significantly reduced compassion fatigue and burnout as measured by the ProQOL (Semerci, et al., 2020). Compared to their peers without training, teachers trained in multiple intervention techniques to address student trauma, including progressive muscle relaxation, report higher levels of performance and self-efficacy in helping students manage emotions and practice coping strategies (Wolmer, et al., 2016).

Practicing gratitude

Gratitude is a two-step process of recognizing a positive outcome, as well as an external source (or sources) for that outcome. Increasing gratitude through deliberate practice is linked to improved health and happiness, as well as stronger relationships (Allen, 2018). Gratitude practices can include:

- Keeping a gratitude journal, such as writing down a set number things for which you are grateful, as well as the causes of those things

- Reflecting on what life could be like if a specific positive event had not occurred
- Spending money on experiences, such as shared meals or concert outings, instead of material goods like clothing or jewelry
- Writing a thank you note and delivering it personally

Gratitude can have dark implications in situations of harm and injustice, especially where compassionate awareness is leveraged to imply that someone should be content or even happy with *relatively* less harm than *could* happen to them. Elevating the expectation of "thanks" or "silver linings" may prioritize tolerance of oppression, imply blame for failing to persevere and minimize or deny serious problems. Gratitude is an effective coping mechanism and often treated as "good for the person and good for society," but it must not come at the expense of disturbance about social injustice, effective resistance and good faith efforts to transform intolerable harm. For students and educators grappling with inequity and injustice, a lack of gratitude "may be a more moral response." Gratitude can also lead to identifying with others who have similar circumstances, luck
or privileges at the expense of others (Jackson, 2016). To address these challenges, trauma-informed educators help students experience and express gratitude in appropriate circumstances and with context (Wong, Cho, & Pandelios, 2024), including:

- **Humility:** The recognition that others' interests and needs are as worthy of concern as one's own
- **Empathy:** Experiencing some of the emotions that another person feels and using social perspective to discern or carefully consider another person's thoughts, emotions and motivations
- **Altruism:** A motivation to help others out of genuine concern for their welfare

Reflections

- How often do you incorporate rhythmic physical activity in your work with students?
- How can you make these other grounding practices part of your routine at school?

Recommended resource

"Greater Good in Education: Science-Based Practices for Kinder, Happier Schools" by the Greater Good Science Center, **ggie.berkeley.edu**

4 Exercise healthy relational boundaries

CONTENT NOTE. This chapter includes ideas related to deficit narrative, drug use and mental illness.

"How should we determine when a supportive relationship with students ends, and a clinical exploration of trauma begins?"

—Alex Shevrin Venet (Role-Clarity and Boundaries for Trauma-Informed Teachers, 2019)

This course focuses on building educators' skills—especially among folks who are not social workers, counselors, psychologists or clinicians, or who are not trained to address mental health. Learning more often leads to wanting to do more and better for students. Yet it's important to understand that when it comes to trauma, some types of "doing more" can cause harm (Barrett, n.d.). For example, this text does not prepare readers to analyze or process trauma narratives.

Being a trauma-informed educator does not require knowing any details of a student's story. Furthermore, *soliciting* trauma narratives—also called being a "trauma detective" (Venet, 2021) and "trauma chasing" (Eklund, Koriakin, Chafouleas, & Dodge, 2020)—can be harmful. For a person with traumatic effects, talking about trauma does not always make it better and can lead to deeply unsettling experiences, like dissociation, flashbacks and re-traumatization.

Deficits and savior mentality

"Saviorism is a pretense at benevolent dominance that freezes its targets into objects, things 'both barbarous and passive, worth rescuing but not freeing,' in the words of Rinaldo Walcott."
—Dionne Brand (Salvage: Readings from the Wreck, 2024)

Learning about the effects of trauma can sometimes sound like highlighting all that can go wrong with students' development. Trauma-informed literature often includes terms, analogies and framing that contribute to the idea that children who have faced adversity are irreparably damaged, broken or bad. Reading or consuming too much from that lens, without critique, can lead to the idea that trauma shifts sociopolitical and historical contexts into personal problems. Deficit views transform into a savior mentality when educators, with positions of power, combine the faulty logic of deficits with good intentions and try to "help" in ways that do not actually help (Venet, 2021).

Operating from a savior mentality looks like neglecting a student's assets and instead elevating our own capacities. It can also include expecting students to express gratitude for good intentions and warm affect. Be vigilant against deficit narratives that situate problems as inherent to a student or their family, rather than as a reasonable response to inputs. Notice and challenge saviorism when it emerges in education. The remainder of this chapter focuses on two key approaches to undermine deficit thinking and savior mentality.

Let go of gratitude as your due

Equity-centered, trauma-informed educators do not aim to heal, fix or save students. Rather, they understand the power of being one of many caring adults in a child's life as essential to health and healing. Becoming a trauma-informed educator means embracing kindness, improving practices for positive psychology and exuding warmth, among other things. We owe students these things as people, because we understand and respect our role in their human development. They do not "owe" us a reciprocal debt of thanks; we should not expect them to "repay" us with preferred attitudes, behaviors or beliefs. Practice expressing gratitude for students' strengths, capacity and potential as a way of inviting authentic, rather than transactional, gratitude into the school community.

Establish healthy boundaries

Students with trauma often have boundary issues; they benefit from educators stating and holding clear boundaries and expectations (Barrett, n.d.; Venet, 2021). Setting and assessing boundaries is not a one-time event. Trauma-informed educators can and should:

- Support students who are struggling to self-regulate on a tough day, feeling sad or angry, or feeling challenged to relate to peers.
- Use authentic relationships and social-emotional engagement strategies.
- Facilitate connections: Build bridges, remove barriers and clear paths between students and supports.
- Reflect on the social and emotional dimensions of your work; identify opportunities to improve your practice, such as by expanding and universalizing accommodations.
- Talk and share generally about how stress and trauma can impact our brains, bodies and behaviors to normalize this science and these realities for students.
- Acknowledge human responses—including strong and unpleasant emotions; introduce and review vocabulary and strategies to label and regulate feelings.

Conversely, most trauma-informed educators should ask for help or make a referral to specialized instructional support personnel (SISP)—such as a school nurse, psychologist or social worker—if an individual student needs:

- Assistance to process traumatic memories in depth
- Acute care during a mental health crisis
- Screening for a behavioral health challenge—including mental illness and substance misuse
- Diagnosis or labeling of an experience and its effects
- Help to create a personalized plan to improve or manage their mental health

Many educators report "time pressure" as a stressor as they struggle to balance many tasks with limited time and resources (AFT, 2015; AFT, 2017). Moreover, working to become more emotionally vulnerable with students and cultivating spaces for psychological safety can make it easier for young people to ask for help with things that exceed your professional skill set or capacity. It is important to set intentions and vocalize boundaries, such as on your time, when your work is overwhelming or leading to unmanageable exposure to violence.

Reflections

- What distinguishes healthy boundaries from callousness, or arbitrary limits on access to your caring?
- (Re)Visit the policy ideas in the section on "Systemic change" in the chapter titled "Elevate educator wellness." Can you think of at least two parallel policy ideas to change schools as institutions in support of student well-being?

Recommended resource

Equity-Centered Trauma-Informed Education by Alex Shevrin Venet

Promote well-being

This section introduces and contextualizes basic science on how trauma affects children's brains, bodies and behaviors. The U.S. Substance Abuse and Mental Health Services Administration's (SAMHSA) 3Es model offers a framework to structure trauma-informed interventions in schools. The 3Es inform the entire CARE-FULL course and especially the next few chapters, including "Develop a lens not a label," "Facilitate post-traumatic growth," "Support grieving students" and "Reduce the risk of abuse."

CARE-FULL focuses on primary prevention, also called Tier 1, universal and schoolwide approaches. Throughout this text, we concentrate on up-to-date evidence that informs skills all educators can use to promote all students' mental health and well-being—whether those students have faced adversity, are diagnosed as having a mental illness or have shared personal details about trauma. These practices are also selected for being extremely helpful and healing for students who are struggling to achieve or maintain well-being. In other words, consistently using these trauma-informed practices supports all students while giving those who need it an extra boost toward wellness.

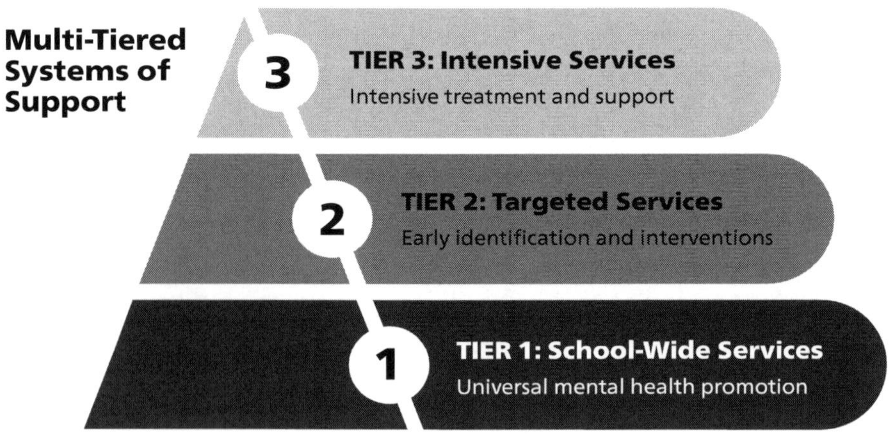

Multi-tiered systems of support rely on increasingly intense interventions to prevent and then address needs and challenges.

"Trauma" is used to name diverse things. The word is used confusingly: as both cause and effect, as something common and rare. In this chapter, we focus on 3Es to navigate this concept: event (exposure, environment) + experience + effect, explained by SAMHSA (Concept of Trauma and Guidance for a Trauma-Informed Approach, 2014).

Traumatic events

> *"Violence is not just a thing that happens between two people. It can be enacted by institutions like the police and hospitals. It is not simply active harm, but blocking access to health and economic security."*
>
> —Vanessa Carlisle (West, 2021)

The first "E" in SAMHSA's model names harmful events, exposures and environments. Children may face direct, indirect, structural and/or historical violence. Exposure to violence is ubiquitous and can be considered a public health epidemic. Furthermore, community instability upsets children's health and development trajectories (Department of Health and Human Services, 2022). Traumatic events may include:

- **Abuse.** Ten percent of U.S. high school students overall reported physical abuse during the coronavirus pandemic. Lesbian, gay and bisexual students were twice as likely to report physical abuse (20 percent) as heterosexual students (10 percent) (Department of Health and Human Services, 2022).
- **Community violence.** As both direct targets and witnesses, community violence is a common childhood experience among 18 percent of youth each year and 28 percent in their lifetime (Rohde-Collins, 2020; Department of Health and Human Services, 2022).
- **Domestic violence.** It's a part of childhood for about 1 in 5 youth overall and more than 1.5 million each year (Phifer, 2020).
- **Food insecurity.** Nearly a third of Black adolescent students reported experiencing it during the coronavirus pandemic (Department of Health and Human Services, 2022).
- **Investigation by child protective services.** Overall this impacts more than 1 in 3 children before the age of 18 and more than every other Black child in the U.S. (Kim, Wildeman, Jonson-Reid, & Drake, 2017).
- **Homelessness.** An estimated 1 in 30 children annually experience it (Bowman & Popp, 2020).
- **Parental incarceration.** This has touched 10 million youth overall and about 2.7 million each year (Sullivan, 2020).
- **Racism.** More than 1 in 3 high school students reported being treated badly or unfairly at school due to race or ethnicity. Asian, Black and multiracial students reported the highest levels of racism (Department of Health and Human Services, 2022).

Traumatic experience

In SAMHSA's 3Es model, the second "E" is for traumatic experience. Humans respond to traumatic events, usually with strong and unpleasant emotions, as well as considerable stress. Just as every physical wound does not become sepsis, not all stress becomes toxic to the point of causing trauma.

A traumatic event becomes a traumatic experience if it overwhelms a young person's coping capacity, causes hard-to-manage emotional and physical responses and generates a sense of being in crisis. Traumatic experiences are common after traumatic events (National Child Traumatic Stress Network Schools Committee, 2008; Jaycox, Langley, & Dean, 2009; Maynard, Farina, Dell, & Kelly, 2019). Traumatic experiences are more likely to occur in the context of chronic and interpersonal adversity than after acute and non-interpersonal events, such as natural disasters or motor vehicle accidents (Blaustein & Kinniburgh, 2019).

Common Traumatic Experiences After Traumatic Events
adapted from (Jaycox, Langley, & Dean, 2009)

Feeling anger. Some people feel angry about the event or about the things that happened afterward. Other people just feel angry all the time, at everything and everybody. Both responses are normal and will get better as you begin to digest what happened to you.

Feeling shame. Sometimes people are ashamed about what happened to them. Sometimes, stress can make you feel bad about yourself, like you're a bad person or that no one likes you. This makes it harder to be friendly and to have fun with others. Even though it's hard to believe, this gets better the more that you talk about what happened. Keeping your feelings a secret makes it more difficult for shame to go away.

Feeling guilt. People can feel guilty about what happened or about something they did or did not do. Sometimes you blame yourself for things that you couldn't control. You may also feel guilty for upsetting others. Guilty feelings can make it hard to talk about what happened.

Feeling sadness, grief or loss. Sometimes stressful or traumatic events include losing someone close to you or losing something that is important to you. This can make you feel sad and down.

Fear, tension and having nightmares or trouble sleeping. After something scary or upsetting, it takes a while to figure out exactly what happened and what it means. After severe stress or traumatic events, people tend to keep thinking about what happened in order to "digest" it, just like your stomach has to work to digest a big meal. This can take a long time. Nightmares are one way of digesting what happened to you.

Feeling afraid for seemingly no reason. This occurs because you remember what happened or because you are thinking about what happened. Other times it occurs because your body is so tense that you start feeling scared.

Anxiety and thinking about it all the time. This is another way to digest what happened. Just like having nightmares, thinking about the traumatic event all the time is a problem because it makes you feel upset. It can be unpleasant.

Avoidance and wanting to NOT think or talk about it. This is natural, since it is upsetting to think about a past stressor and doing so can lead to diverse emotions. Avoidance makes things easier, but only for a little while. Avoiding situations that remind you of what happened can help you feel better right then. But avoidance may keep you from doing normal things that are an important part of your life. It's important to digest what happened sooner or later.

Vigilance and being on guard to protect yourself; feeling like something bad is about to happen. After something bad happens to you, it makes sense to be prepared for another bad thing. But you can spend so much time waiting for the next bad thing to happen that you don't have time or energy for other things in your life. Also, it is scary to think something bad is going to happen.

Not being able to remember parts of what happened. Stressful events can be so awful that your memory doesn't work as usual. Sometimes it gets easier to remember later on and sometimes it gets harder. This can be frustrating, but it is normal.

Having trouble concentrating. With the nervousness you are feeling and all the time you are spending thinking about what happened, it can be hard to concentrate on work or even on what your friends or family say to you.

Jumping when there is a loud noise. This is one way that your body says it is prepared for action in case something else happens. As you begin to feel calmer, this will go away.

Having physical health problems and complaints. Stress affects your body as well. People sometimes get sick more often or notice pain and discomfort more often when they have been under stress.

Feeling out of control. If a lot of these common reactions are problems for you, you can start to feel out of control or even "crazy." Don't worry, though; they are all normal reactions and there are ways to help you feel better.

This list should be used for awareness and understanding. Screening students for traumatic effects and labeling or diagnosing for related conditions or illnesses are the responsibilities of clinicians and not covered in this text.

Many of these traumatic experiences or trauma responses are also on the lists of indicators of common mental illnesses after a crisis event—researchers especially look for signs of post-traumatic stress disorder (PTSD), depression and anxiety. The difference between a traumatic experience and a high risk of developing traumatic effects, or an altered developmental trajectory, is usually intensity of exposure and time.

Traumatic effects

The third "E" in SAMHSA's model is for traumatic effects. Traumatic exposure and traumatic experiences cause significant stress in the body. Left unchecked, the body's stress response can become toxic to developing internal systems. High levels of the hormone cortisol can especially wreak havoc. If young people are excessively exposed to unmitigated traumatic events and cannot cope, they can develop traumatic effects, or persistent changes to their brains, bodies and behaviors. Traumatic effects that may appear in school can include:

- Struggle with executive functions (focus, logically sequence, organize, plan, problem-solve, process information, set and follow through with goals), expressive language, as well as emotional regulation
- Poor performance on academic assessments, standardized state assessments, language tasks and IQ tests
- School avoidance and missed institutional milestones: failing a grade, repeating a grade, chronic absenteeism, dropping out
- Low self-esteem, social withdrawal
- Exclusion from instruction and/or school through suspension or expulsion

> Eliminating childhood trauma could reduce some adult health issues by up to
> **44%**
> (Merrick, et al., 2019).

Stigmatizing labels such as "hyperactive, aggressive, oppositional and noncompliant," as well as referral to special education, can seem to define students by their struggles. Reframing encourages a focus on the whole student, including attention to possible reasons for challenging behaviors.

Over the course of a lifetime, traumatic events show a dose-response relationship with poor health outcomes in adulthood. In other words, for every additional adverse exposure, a person's risk of traumatic effects increases (Pfeffer, 2018). High incidence of childhood adversity is linked to adults who are more likely to do all of the following (Merrick, et al., 2019; Centers for Disease Control and Prevention, 2019):

- Adopt behaviors that increase risks for poor health outcomes, such as alcohol abuse, illicit drug use and smoking
- Experience asthma, cancer, depression, diabetes, heart disease, intimate partner violence, kidney disease, suicide attempts
- Experience elevated rates of cell and tissue damage and death, inflammation and poor health
- Pass higher likelihood of poor health outcomes to their children epigenetically; model ineffective coping strategies

In sum, exposure to violence increases children's likelihood of developing long-term changes (Substance Abuse and Mental Health Services Administration, 2014). One study estimates that eliminating adverse child experiences could reduce some adult health issues by up to 44 percent (Merrick, et al., 2019). Traumatic events can shift child development, including the composition of neural networks related to language, memory and attachment; gene expression; chromosomal replication; and stress reactivity (Centers for Disease Control and Prevention, 2019). In simple terms, children who face adversity are more likely to struggle with communicating, participating in trusting relationships, concentrating and staying calm. They are also more likely to excel at survival behaviors that feel at odds with traditional learning environments and academic expectations.

The 3Es model is exciting for trauma-informed educators because it clarifies multiple meaningful points of intervention for student wellness. These points of intervention can occur before students experience unnecessary adversity, before a traumatic event becomes a traumatic experience and before a traumatic experience becomes lasting traumatic effects. Read on to learn more about how you can facilitate health and healing with attention to these opportunities.

5 Develop a lens, not a label

CONTENT NOTE. This chapter includes ideas related to colonialism and racism.

> *"Once we identify our students who struggle, how can we help them heal and develop in ways that will set them up for success? Can we focus on our students' strengths rather than their deficits? Can we view our students as overflowing with potential rather than doomed to failure? It's up to us."*
>
> —Kristin Souers and Pete Hall (Fostering Resilient Learners: Strategies for Creating a Trauma-Sensitive Classroom, 2016)

Trauma-informed educators understand that each "E" in SAMHSA's model—traumatic event, traumatic experience and traumatic effect—poses an opportunity for intervention. Making time to learn about students does not mean that you require them to disclose sensitive information or "perform poverty;" learning about students should not turn you into a "trauma detective" (Venet, 2021). Trauma-informed educators endeavor to bring the same lens to all interactions—with students, colleagues and families.

A student's race, gender, class and other social identities shape their experiences with trauma as well as their coping strategies. For instance, Black and Indigenous students may endure not only personal trauma but also collective and historical trauma from racism and colonialism. Trauma-informed educators must consider these intersections to offer equitable supports that address each student's unique experience—or strategically remove unnecessary barriers altogether.

Unconditional positive regard

In 1957, Carl Rogers declared unconditional positive regard to be one of six essential conditions for psychological healing. He explained, "It means there are no conditions of acceptance, no feeling of 'I like you only if you are thus and so ...'" (Rogers C. , 1957). His therapeutic approach honored and centered the person who was hurting. He further encouraged therapists to think of themselves as facilitators rather than experts, sharing power rather than exercising it over clients (Edwards B. , 2021). Rogers' ideas have been adapted for education and often appear in trauma-informed education models (Brunzell, Stokes, & Waters, 2019; Hertel & Johnson, 2020; Venet, 2021).

Educators intuitively and perhaps even unanimously endorse positive relationships as central to success with students. Yet forming healthy bonds and maintaining unconditional positive regard can be challenging, especially with students who resist educators' efforts to be in a relationship (Brunzell, Stokes, & Waters, 2019). Unconditional positive regard means that students are accepted for who they are—not based on their performance or compliance. It requires seeing students as their own people with unique strengths. Unconditional positive regard means that any educator could say to any of the students they serve:

> *"You know what? I really, really like you. You can keep doing all this stuff and it's not going to change my mind. It seems to me that you are trying to get me to dislike you, but it's not going to work. I'm not ever going to do that" (Watson & Ecken, 2003).*

Learn more about how to show unconditional positive regard with the healing gestures in the chapter titled, "Facilitate positive experiences."

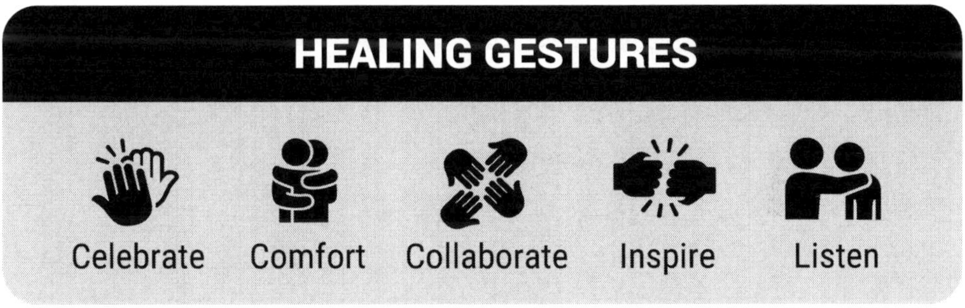

Five healing gestures in the national Changing Minds Now campaign (Futures Without Violence, 2024).

Reflections

- Write out your beliefs, intentions and guiding questions—your lens—as a trauma-informed educator
- What is your next organic opportunity to learn more about students' gifts, talents and strengths?

Recommended resource

"Concept of Trauma and Guidance for a Trauma-Informed Approach," by the Substance Abuse and Mental Health Services Administration, U.S. Department of Health and Human Services, **store.samhsa.gov/product/SAMHSA-s-Concept-of-Trauma-and-Guidance-for-a-Trauma-Informed-Approach/SMA14-4884.html**

6 Facilitate post-traumatic growth

CONTENT NOTE. This chapter includes ideas related to deficit narrative and mental illness.

> *"Many people develop specialized abilities because of exposures to adversity."*
>
> —Ellis et al. (Hidden Talents in Harsh Environments, 2020)

A lot of mainstream messaging about trauma focuses on deficits and undesirable outcomes; words like "damage," "dysregulation" and "disorder" are common. However, trauma can also uniquely catalyze growth and push adaptive strengths. Attending to these positive possibilities and how to nurture them is an important part of healing-centered engagement and recognizing the dignity of people who have faced adversity. This chapter focuses on educators' role in supporting post-traumatic growth, which is characterized by five changes (Gendre, Soubelet, & Callahan, 2024):

- **Appreciation for life:** getting more out of life, feeling lucky to be alive
- **Relationships with others:** experiencing interpersonal connections as more intimate, more deeply appreciated or more compassionate
- **Developing personal strength:** feeling more capable or resilient and able to face difficulties
- **New possibilities:** trying out novel behaviors and activities
- **Spiritual development:** considering big picture questions about life and existence, as well as rethinking one's beliefs

Other researchers summarize post-traumatic growth more succinctly as increased self-esteem and positive relationships (Mangelsdorf, Eid, & Luhmann, 2018). Such growth reflects a struggle after trauma to (re)evaluate one's goals, beliefs and worldview. Post-traumatic growth may exist alongside post-traumatic stress, including symptoms that meet the criteria for a diagnosis for PTSD (Vloet, Vloet, Bürger, & Romanos, 2017).

Post-traumatic growth is dynamic

Post-traumatic growth, significant positive change due to exposure to a traumatic event, is more than the absence of symptoms or return to baseline functioning (Bernstein & Pfefferbaum, 2018). Such growth is not stable or easy to chart. Rather than a "straight line" from traumatic event to growth (or struggles with traumatic effects), most individuals experience complex journeys. Indeed, post-traumatic journeys often include signs of significant distress, false starts, setbacks and illusory highs (Gendre, Soubelet, & Callahan, 2024). We can simplify post-traumatic journeys into three broad profiles or "types." After a traumatic event:

- About three in 10 students are resilient and quick to recover: They exhibit low signs of post-traumatic stress and quickly return to baseline levels of coping and symptomology. If these students already had mental illness, such as anxiety or depression, their symptoms will be unchanged—neither better nor worse (Bernstein & Pfefferbaum, 2018).
- About half of students undergo a prolonged, up-and-down journey to post-traumatic growth and recovery. These students show elevated challenges for up to 12 months yet also develop long-lasting new strengths and capacities (Bernstein & Pfefferbaum, 2018; Xiaoli, et al., 2019). In fact, moderate symptoms of PTSD predict high post-traumatic growth (Gendre, Soubelet, & Callahan, 2024).
- About one in 5 students struggle with persistent traumatic effects, including severe, ongoing psychological symptoms and signs of post-traumatic stress disorder (Bernstein & Pfefferbaum, 2018).

50%

About half of students experience an up-and-down journey for the 12 months after a traumatic event that ends in post-traumatic growth and recovery.

About two years after a traumatic event, a person's growth and challenges are likely to be settled (Gendre, Soubelet, & Callahan, 2024). However, a student's long-term struggle is not necessarily a cause for hopelessness; some children take more than five years to achieve post-traumatic growth (Mangelsdorf, Eid, & Luhmann, 2018).

Several factors influence an individual's post-traumatic journey. For example, older children tend to experience more growth, while younger children are more likely to develop persistent symptoms of disorder (Gendre, Soubelet, & Callahan, 2024). The level of exposure to the traumatic event also matters; repeated exposure and more direct exposure are both associated with greater traumatic effects (Bernstein & Pfefferbaum, 2018). Access to social support, especially over time, is a particularly potent predictor of whether a traumatic event will persist in traumatic effects (Blaustein & Kinniburgh, 2019). Secondary losses, or changes that ripple around a child after a traumatic event, also impact outcomes. The more "ripples" a traumatic event causes, the more likely a young person is to face higher risk for mental illness (Schonfeld & Quackenbush, 2021).

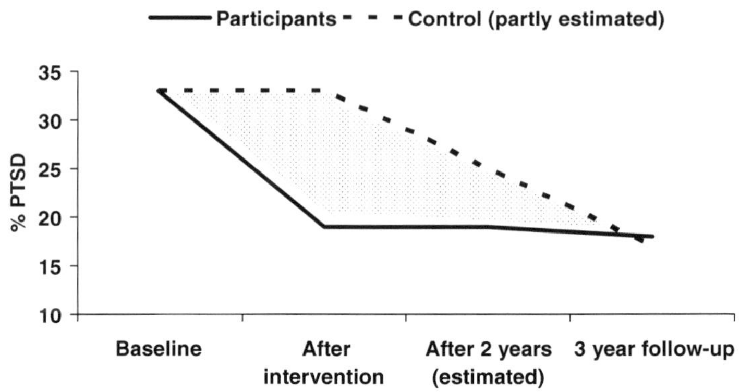

Three-year estimates of post-traumatic stress disorder rates in children who participated in a school-based trauma intervention compared to a control group. Trauma-informed educators can reduce post-traumatic stress symptoms faster than students would otherwise recover (Wolmer, Laor, Dedeoglu, Siev, & Yazgan, 2005).

Leverage plasticity

In students, the dynamism of post-traumatic growth trajectories after a traumatic event reflects the profound plasticity—or openness to change—of the youthful brain (Wenger & Kühn, 2021). The same plasticity is precisely what makes school-based trauma-informed interventions so potentially powerful. Schools that implement interventions by trained staff may help children resolve PTSD symptoms faster than schools that conduct no intervention (Wolmer, Laor, Dedeoglu, Siev, & Yazgan, 2005).

Help students make meaning

Post-traumatic growth is the outcome of grappling with a traumatic event and its implications—and ultimately developing new strengths and skills to leverage protective factors. Thinking about a traumatic event and its effects is often initially intrusive and seemingly out-of-control. Learning to deliberately, rather than reflexively, reflect on traumatic events helps young people establish new narratives and realize that acknowledging a harm does not automatically replicate its effects (Bernstein & Pfefferbaum, 2018; Jaycox, Langley, & Dean, 2009; Gendre, Soubelet, & Callahan, 2024). Trauma-informed educators try to help students iteratively ruminate toward growth, with prompts such as:

- Have you learned anything as a result of this experience?
- Can you find meaning in this experience?
- Does anything help you accept that this has happened?

Importantly, making space for realizations is not the same as requiring the discovery of silver linings. Opportunities to practice toward post-traumatic growth do not demand an end to that growth process or punish or abandon students for exhibiting a "rollercoaster" of emotions or traumatic responses. Rather, trauma-informed educators can assist students in strengthening skills for resilience, such as identifying their assets and asking for help.

Coordinate peer support

Improved social relationships are an essential element of post-traumatic growth (Mangelsdorf, Eid, & Luhmann, 2018; Gendre, Soubelet, & Callahan, 2024). In addition to practicing healing gestures and other capacities to be safe, stable and nurturing presences in students' lives, trauma-informed educators prepare students to support each other (Schonfeld & Quackenbush, 2021). Students are more likely to practice empathy when it is effectively and regularly modeled in their school community. Furthermore, students benefit from direct instruction about the basic facts of trauma.

Recenter learning around hidden talents

> *"Successful adaptation may manifest in many ways, and often in ways that seem counterintuitive. For instance, a child who is labeled manipulative and a liar (common descriptors of a neglected child) is often a child who has successfully adapted to a world in which needs are not met by finding ways to meet those needs. A child who appears emotionally shut down may be a child who has successfully adapted to a failure of caretaking by minimizing access to emotional experience."*
> *—Blaustein and Kinniburgh (Treating Traumatic Stress in Children and Adolescents: How to Foster Resilience through Attachment, Self-Regulation, and Competency, 2019)*

Traumatized students are often exquisitely attuned for success ... albeit in circumstances very different from those we strive to create for learning. The hidden talents framework focuses on social and cognitive skills that develop in response to adversity (Ellis, et al., 2020), such as:

- Collaborative contributions to collective outcomes
- Decoding nonverbal cues
- Detecting changes in dynamic visual information
- Extracting resources and rewards from unpredictable environments
- High compassion and attentiveness to others' needs
- Identifying deceit
- Rapidly and accurately detecting anger and possible aggressive stimuli (e.g., weapons)
- Strong attunement to social information and social relationships, in other words, high sensitivity to human power dynamics

Importantly, research suggests that educators who plan learning experiences to leverage hidden talents can "unlock" unique, stress-adapted skills. For example, students who have faced complex and compounded adversity may be great leaders under pressure (Foo, 2022). Educators should consider how lessons or interventions can (Ellis, et al., 2020):

- Discuss status, rank and power.
- Identify and build on prior knowledge.
- Increase collaboration rather than competition.
- Increase measurement against a generic standard rather than measurement against peers.
- Introduce and assess skills using project-based learning grounded in students' cultural and ecological context.
- Require attention shifting and complex tracking: use background noise, regularly change focus, display content on dynamic touch screens, apply skills in changing contexts, provide real-time feedback on tasks or performance.

Reflections

- Which part of this chapter is most surprising to you? Which part is most familiar?
- Of the three strategies offered in this chapter to hasten post-traumatic growth—help students make meaning, coordinate peer support and recenter learning around hidden talents—which are you likely to try first?

Recommended resource

"Student Stories of Pandemic Trauma" by Jim Arey and Chelsea Prax, **aftvoices.org/student-stories-of-pandemic-trauma-bbc089604cd1**

7 Support grieving students

CONTENT NOTE. This chapter includes ideas related to coronavirus pandemic, death, drug use, grief, gun violence, racism and suicide.

> *"Who knows what the right language, the right behavior, the right sounds you're supposed to make—to show that you're considerate, sensitive, compassionate, sympathetic. [We act as though] to be the most indirect you can be is to be the most sympathetic—but that is a recipe for the most absolute illiteracy where dying is concerned."*
>
> —Stephen Jenkinson (Orphan Wisdom, 2014)

In 2009, the AFT and New York Life Foundation partnered to survey educators. Two striking findings—that most educators felt unprepared to support grieving students and that they were eager to participate in professional development—inspired the creation of the Coalition to Support Grieving Students (Densen, Lansworth, & Siegel, 2012). Convened by the National Center for School Crisis and Bereavement, the coalition brings together over 100 organizations that represent teachers, counselors, nurses, psychologists, principals, superintendents, bereavement experts and more. Coalition members develop and promote free, high-quality resources focused on making schools and educators grief-sensitive. More recent research shows educators remain committed to providing grief support and continue to have a strong interest in training (AFT & New York Life Foundation, 2020).

According to a joint survey by AFT and New York Life Foundation (2020):

93% Nearly all educators (93%) agreed that childhood grief is a serious problem that deserves more attention from schools.

87% Most educators (87%) said that at least one student each year typically needs their support due to the loss of a loved one.

This chapter covers and builds upon content from the Coalition to Support Grieving Students.

In 2022,
1,089
children in the United States were newly bereaved each day.

Snapshot of Child Bereavement Estimation Model (CBEM) results derived from current analyses, judishouse.wpengine.com/research-tools/cbem/.

Grief at school

By age 18, 13.7 percent of children face the death of a parent or sibling (Childhood Bereavement Estimation Model, 2024). In 2022, over one thousand children were newly bereaved each day (Childhood Bereavement Estimation Model, 2024).

Most grief does not lead to traumatic effects; still, it impacts learning and can pose challenges at school, especially for students who do not receive appropriate accommodations. Immediately following a death, in families where adults are busy with preparations and logistics, students may face reduced family supervision, which can in turn lead to changes in the submission of assignments and study habits. Grieving students are often distracted and struggle to concentrate; during periods of acute bereavement, this may result in challenges with taking in or remembering new concepts and facts. Finally, mourning students who had preexisting challenges with learning may show reduced academic performance if they are not accommodated (Schonfeld & Quackenbush, 2021).

Challenge the silence

It is normal and common for young people to grieve, yet many cultures have strong taboos against talking about death. We tend to believe that talking about death is inappropriate, rude, blunt or possibly harmful (Orphan Wisdom, 2014). Likewise, we rarely use the words "death" or "die" and instead use euphemisms such as "loss," "passed," "kicked the bucket" and "final resting place." These kinds of oblique references contribute to communication challenges and confusion among grieving students (Orphan Wisdom, 2014).

Children often misunderstand or incompletely understand death and loss, as well as related circumstances and responses. They may misread adult responses, such as looking away or not continuing a conversation and crying. For example, children may conclude they have done something wrong by talking about death and avoid raising the subject again. They may also suppress feelings and try to look fine to support families when they need support. Finally, bereaved young people often feel overwhelmed by the experience and may have trouble expressing complicated feelings (Schonfeld & Quackenbush, 2021).

Students appreciate emotional space and support to talk about death. Even if adults are uncomfortable, students benefit from them guiding dialogue with the following key principles:

- **Be present.** Assume that while death is upsetting, talking about it is not. On the contrary, not acknowledging bereavement or saying nothing is the wrong thing.
- **Initiate a conversation.** Express concern, ask open-ended questions and offer to connect privately or arrange connections to another adult.
- **Listen more than you talk.** Express genuine sympathy and empathy. Avoid sharing personal stories. Share nonjudgmental observations about behavior and responses. Avoid attempts to "cheer up" or alleviate the pain.
- **Offer emotional space.** All children benefit from dedicated time to grieve, talk about death and learn new ways to communicate. Identify opportunities for healthy emotional expression with practical advice. Stop harmful or dangerous behaviors. Maintain contact and long-term reassurance, as appropriate.

Trauma-informed educators develop and foster death literacy and learn to be direct and clear. In preparing to be open and straightforward about grief and loss, consider four universal truths about death that apply no matter a child's cultural, linguistic or developmental status (Schonfeld & Quackenbush, 2021):

- Death is universal. Everything that is alive eventually dies.
- Death is permanent and irreversible.
- Death is final. All life functions end completely at the time of death.
- Death has many possible causes.

Accommodate grieving students

A trauma-informed educator acknowledges unpleasant and difficult emotions and helps students identify ways to manage them. While it can be difficult to choose simple presence when someone is distressed, sometimes establishing psychological safety means allowing someone to move through an unpleasant emotion in their own way and at their own pace, instead of trying to transform their emotion into one that is more comfortable. A grief-sensitive educator also offers academic support so that academic demands do not exceed the student's capacity to learn, thereby turning school into another stressor.

Anticipate and manage grief triggers. Over time, grieving usually becomes less intense in the day-to-day. However, grief triggers can return a young person to the powerful emotions that accompany acute bereavement. A grief trigger is a sudden reminder of loss. Common grief triggers include listening to a song, hearing information on the news and certain smells and sounds.

The death of a loved one is considered a primary loss. Secondary losses, the changes that ripple around a child after a death or in the wake of significantly changed life circumstances, are also common grief triggers and can exacerbate the primary loss or death. These include:

- Shifts in relationships, schools, future plans, lifestyle or peer group/status
- A parent who is less available
- Loss of shared memories, special recognition and/or support
- Missed opportunities to share milestones, special occasions and proud moments—such as recitals, sporting activities and parent-specific dances or prom
- Financial challenges
- Decreased sense of security and safety

To plan for grief triggers, trauma-informed educators note special occasions in which the absence of loved ones might suddenly set off a more intense grief response. During birthdays, holidays and days dedicated to parents, even students whose loss is considerably past may appreciate meaningful accommodations. This may look like structured opportunities to share and celebrate memories of the deceased.

Assign appropriate and achievable work. Grieving students benefit from meaningful flexibility that balances high expectations with compassion for changed circumstances, as well as heightened emotionality. Grief-sensitive educators can consider adapting:

- Content focus, including avoiding the exact or very similar circumstances of a child's bereavement
- Format, such as group, partner or individual work and written, typed or recorded submissions
- Pacing, such as by postponing assignments, rescheduling tasks or providing extra time
- Timing, such as to postpone a deadline, shift the number of steps required to show mastery or provide extra time to complete an assessment in a quiet location
- Value or weight of specific assignments, such as by exempting grieving students immediately after a death, as well as omitting or reweighting some scores for final grades

Use a team approach. Grief-sensitive educators can partner with both caregivers and colleagues to better meet the needs of bereaved students. To help students make meaning of the changes that follow a loss, it may be helpful to start an open dialogue with families. Try open-ended questions such as "What have you told your child? What does she understand? What does he misunderstand? Does your family have rituals, traditions or patterns related to the change?"

Grief is a compelling example of a common traumatic event that rarely develops into traumatic effects, or what clinicians call "complicated grief." Still, if grief interferes with a child's learning for weeks without improvement or if they show persistent signs of hopelessness and agitation, it may be time to ask for help from a specialist. Local bereavement organizations and specialized instructional support personnel (SISP)—including school counselors, nurses, social workers and psychologists—may be instrumental if a student's experience becomes worrisome. They may also help classroom and grade-specific educators to compile and share information through a student's transitions, such as to a new grade or new school.

Childhood grief reveals national patterns of inequity

Not all children are equally likely to be burdened with grief. Indigenous and Black children are more likely than other kids to be bereaved by age 18. Furthermore, they are much more likely to grapple with the death of parents due to preventable diseases like cancer, diabetes and heart disease (Childhood Bereavement Estimation Model, 2021).

Widespread public health crises exacerbate existing equity challenges. For example, in the first two years of the coronavirus pandemic hundreds of thousands of children became newly bereaved due to increases in deaths related to novel coronavirus disease (a cause of more than 1 in 10 parent deaths), as well as parent deaths by increased rates of accidental overdose, homicide by gunshot and suicide (Childhood Bereavement Estimation Model, 2023; Burns, et al., 2023). These grim statistics highlight the fact that grief is related to systemic oppression, including because of select divestment, inequitable access to healthcare and failures to protect marginalized communities. Further, such "stigmatized losses may result in increased isolation, guilt and uncertainty for grieving families" (Burns, et al., 2023). Trauma-informed educators who work with students burdened by layered bereavement have unique opportunities to guide critical reflection on the social conditions that disparately distribute mourning, as well as how loving political action may shift conditions—or at least aid healing (Táíwò O. , 2022; Ginwright, 2018; Gross, 2024).

Reflections

Develop your own "go-to" phrases and questions for speaking with a grieving student.

Recommended resource

The Coalition to Support Grieving Students, **grievingstudents.org**

8 Reduce the risk of abuse

CONTENT NOTE. This chapter includes ideas related to classism, family separation, maltreatment, mental illness and racism.

> *"Poverty, lack of material resources, and other forms of 'imperfect' parenting should not prompt coercive intervention by child welfare agencies or police."*
>
> —Mical Raz (Abusive Policies: How the American Child Welfare System Lost Its Way, 2020)

Like other traumatic events, child maltreatment can lead to traumatic effects, including hypervigilance, disrupted relationships, regularly dysregulated emotional states and significant struggles at school—including low academic performance and increased risk of punishment (Weegar, 2019). Unlike other traumatic events, child maltreatment is the focus of laws in all 50 states that push educators toward a single intervention: reporting to child protective services (CPS). This chapter reviews the effects of mandatory reporting as well as the evidence for more effective school-based strategies to prevent and address child abuse and neglect.

Status quo

Violence against children can take many forms. Child protective services agencies are generally concerned with just three: physical abuse, sexual abuse and neglect. Since the 1960s, child protective services agencies have depended on mandatory reporters to investigate child maltreatment. Despite being some of the nation's most active mandatory reporters—making every fifth report or about 885,000 in 2022—educators rarely understand what happens next (Children's Bureau, 2024).

1. **Screening:** After receiving a report, CPS conducts a screening to determine whether it will follow up. About half of all referrals are declined. Though "screened out" families rarely receive services, they are often placed on a watchlist for monitoring (Baughman, Coles, Feinberg, & Newton, 2021; Slack & Berger, 2020).

2. **Investigation:** Families who are "screened in" undergo an investigation, which is often intrusive, costly and traumatic (Pac, et al., 2023). CPS

caseworkers, sometimes with police, scrutinize every aspect of a family's home and circumstances—including furniture, food, underwear drawers, kitchen cabinets and children's unclothed bodies— regardless of the nature of the report (Roberts, 2022; JMACForFamilies, 2024). Sadly, this is a shockingly common childhood experience; every third U.S. child is subjected to a maltreatment investigation before age 18 (Palmer, Font, Rebbe, & Putnam-Hornstein, 2023).

3. **Determination:** A caseworker's impressions during an investigation are used to label children as either *victims* or *nonvictims* and to establish next steps, which might include required training or counseling, changes to household routines or family separation. Every fifth child in a confirmed case of maltreatment enters foster care (Children's Bureau, 2024).

More sorry than safe

Training and state legislation routinely highlight reporting as the best and only intervention to address child maltreatment (Pietrantoni, Chitiyo, Chitiyo, Peña, & Fernandez, 2023; Raz, 2020). Better understanding the duty to report and how to report does not improve accuracy: Just 10 percent of educators' reports are verified (Children's Bureau, 2024; Baughman, Coles, Feinberg, & Newton, 2021; Walsh, et al., 2022). In other words, up to 9 in 10 times, educators' reports to CPS are not necessary. Instead, reporting may do more harm than good (Crittenden & Spieker, 2023; Itzkowitz & Olson, 2022; Trivedi S. , 2019).

Educators shared the following indicators as prompting their most recent report to CPS:

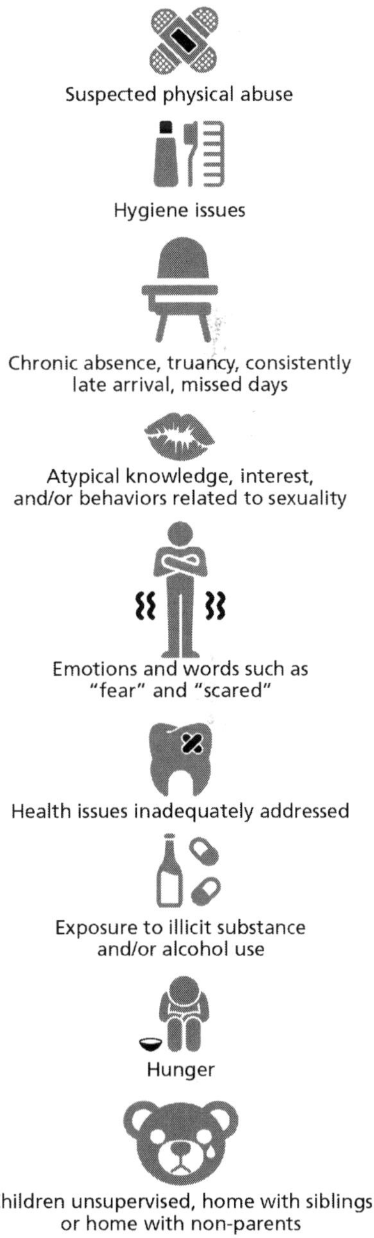

Nine common concerns prompt most of educators' reports to child protective services (Prax, 2025).

Just 10%

of educators' reports to Child Protective Services are verified

(Children's Bureau, 2024; Baughman, Coles, Feinberg, & Newton, 2021; Walsh, et al., 2022).

Reporting and other CPS interventions do not consistently reduce severe injury, child abuse or other forms of maltreatment and often catalyze different harms (Raz, 2020; Russell, Kerwin, & Halverson, 2018). Reporting invokes state agents to enforce normative parental behaviors and control individual caregivers (Raz, 2020; Roberts, 2022). CPS has blunt instruments for engaging system-involved children and families: surveillance, investigation, monitoring, coercion and even family separation (Fong, 2023; Pac, et al., 2023; Roberts, 2022; Children's Bureau, 2024). The agency often agitates, rather than assists, families. System-engaged families quickly become "government averse" and avoid helpers—including educators, healthcare professionals and other social service providers—out of a general distrust that their problems will be adequately or fairly addressed (Fong, 2023). In the words of one former caseworker, CPS "seemed only to manipulate, divide, or subtract. CPS could derail a life [...] The remedial pathways we took often created more complications for families" (Pryce, 2024). Youth involved in CPS are more likely than peers to struggle with mental illness, difficulty in school and unhappiness, leading researchers to conclude, "We found no evidence that contact with the child welfare system improves child outcomes. Rather, CPS contact was associated with worse mental health and developmental outcomes" (Evangelist, Thomas, & Waldfogel, 2023). Educators echo these concerns and often see no improvements or severed relationships after making a report (Prax, 2025).

With 26 times the federal funding for foster care than for maltreatment prevention, CPS often orchestrates child removal into placements where kids face worse risks and outcomes than they did at home (Stoltzfus, 2024; Detlaff, et al., 2020; Sankaran, Church, & Mitchell, 2019). Children in government-coordinated placements have the same poor educational outcomes associated with maltreatment: poor attendance, as well as low academic engagement and attainment (Gypen, Vanderfaeillie, De Maeyer, Belenger, & Van Holen, 2017; Barth, et al., 2020). Furthermore, whereas children often come to the attention of CPS for neglect, in foster care, they are more likely to experience sexual and physical abuse, as well as homelessness and lack of access to healthcare, than they did with their families (Detlaff, et al., 2020). Family separation is "universally negative" for children (Crittenden & Spieker, 2023).

How did we get here?

Educators' rates of reporting have been rising for decades while accuracy rates decline (Krase, 2013; Children's Bureau, 2024). Researchers and workers within the system have known for decades that CPS fails to achieve its mandates (Raz, 2020). Several issues crash together to facilitate these poor outcomes.

Fear drives overreporting (Institute to Transform Child Protection, 2025). Educators fear the loss of professional standing and licensure. CPS workers fear appearing in the news as having failed even one child in serious need (Raz, 2020). Parents often acquiesce to CPS out of a deep fear that their children will be taken from them—an outcome that occurs with stunning regularity anyway: "On any given day, foster care rates for U.S. children, at 563 per 100,000, exceed imprisonment rates for U.S. adults, at 539 per 100,000" (Fong, 2023).

Ambiguity is a hallmark of many components of child maltreatment. Neglect is the most commonly reported type—constituting around three out of four reports—and can be difficult to differentiate from poverty (Children's Bureau, 2024; Itzkowitz & Olson, 2023; Palmer, Font, Eastman, Guo, & Putnam-Hornstein, 2024). About half of the leading concerns educators say prompt their reports to CPS are poverty indicators, including hygiene challenges, chronic absenteeism, health issues, hunger and lack of adult supervision (Prax, 2025). Neglect is also perhaps the most elastic component of maltreatment, easily modified with adjectives like "educational," "emotional" and "medical" to create fluid categories that are hard to research (Prax & Acosta Price, 2025). Broad and vague definitions, combined with sprawling lists of indicators, generally lead to bias, arbitrary decision-making, reduced parental discretion and increased government regulation of families (Raz, 2020).

Poverty is clearly associated with CPS engagement and easy to reframe as neglect, warping a social reality about the inequitable distribution of wealth into a parent's failure to overcome it. Up to 75 percent of verified maltreatment cases are for neglect (Children's Bureau, 2024; Palmer, Font, Eastman, Guo, & Putnam-Hornstein, 2024). Some of the most promising interventions to reduce child maltreatment provide material support to families (Kim & Drake, 2018; Cusick, et al., 2024). However, CPS usually focuses on parenting, such as a caregiver's expectations of their child, capacity to empathize and use of punishment (Fong, 2023; DePanfilis, 2018). These assessments of parents' behavior are at the expense of attention to behavioral influences, including the stress of poverty (U.S. Surgeon General, 2024). Furthermore, outcomes labeled as neglect may better reflect structural rather than parental failures—and therefore require completely different interventions than those CPS is designed to deliver.

Bias—whether conscious or implicit—haunts CPS' work at every stage (Institute to Transform Child Protection, 2025). From referral to investigation and traumatic intervention, children from marginalized groups are overrepresented in CPS' work. This goes beyond the classism we might expect in a system that almost exclusively engages low-income people. Children and parents with disabilities are more likely to be surveilled. Black children are more likely to be investigated. Indigenous families are more likely to be separated (Kim, Wildeman, Jonson-Reid, & Drake, 2017; Merkel-Holguin, et al., 2022; Palusci & Botash, 2021). These disparities are not because disabled, Black or Indigenous people are more likely to be bad parents—but because they are less likely to get necessary support and more likely to be criminalized and punished for struggling.

Respond, rather than react

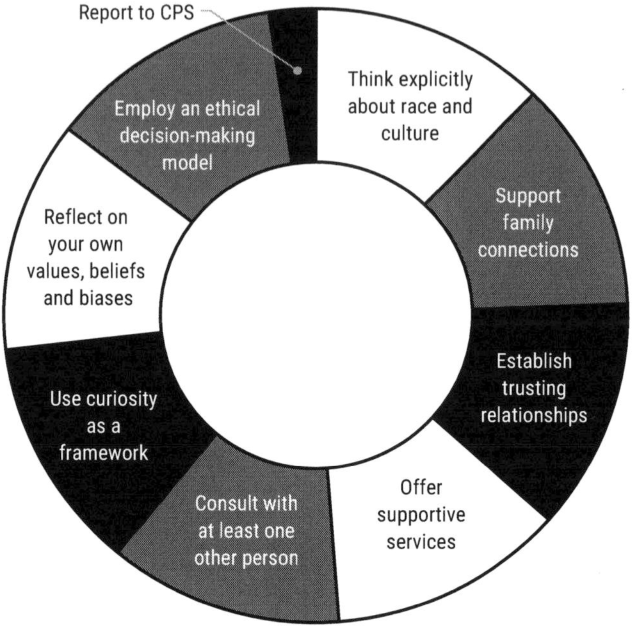

Reporting is one possible response among many to serious concerns about a child's well-being (Itzkowitz & Olson, 2023).

Elevating reporting comes at the expense of preparing educators to effectively prevent maltreatment—or to meaningfully respond to students and families. Families who struggle with child abuse and neglect are often grappling with the stress of compounded challenges that have accrued over time, including barriers to healthcare while managing chronic and mental illnesses, economic strains related to poverty, relocations, divorce and job changes (Fortin, Kwon, & Pierce, 2016; U.S. Surgeon General, 2024; Institute to Transform Child Protection, 2025; Palmer, Font, Eastman, Guo, & Putnam-Hornstein, 2024). For each adversity they face at home, students' risk of suspension and expulsion increases by 80 percent at school (Zeng, Corr, O'Grady, & Guan, 2019). Trauma-informed educators upend this dynamic, increasing support and connections to students and families who show signs of significant stress.

Help caregivers experience confidence: Trauma-informed educators prepare families for success (van der Put, Assink, Gubbels, & van Solinge, 2021).

- Affirm warm and involved caregiving, wherever it takes place and whether the supportive adult is a parent.
- Help families practice strong communication, such as by sharing suggested questions related to school activities that caregivers can use to reinforce learning. Consider structuring chances for students to show evidence of thoughtful connections with family members into learning, such as assigned interviews or extra credit for showing evidence of collaboration, like multiple handwriting samples or signatures.

Within reciprocal and trusting relationships, trauma-informed educators and schools can support families to create safe environments that deter abuse (Rudolph & Zimmer-Gembeck, 2018).

- For families that struggle with childcare or supervision, whether due to conflicts with work schedules or challenges related to health issues, advocate for and streamline connections to out-of-school programming.
- Family engagement programs offer practical opportunities to improve parents' readiness to tackle taboo topics—such as child abuse and youth substance abuse. For example, to increase adults' vigilance against child sexual abuse, a PTA meeting could be dedicated to developing questions to ask of babysitters, neighbors or others who spend time alone with their children (Wortley, Leclerc, Reynald, & Smallbone, 2019).
- As another example, families and educators could collaborate with young people about the best ways to identify and spread fact-based (rather than fear-based) information about illicit substances to maximize well-being (Prax, Paxson, Mandle, & Marcy, 2025).

Start with families: When educators observe indicators that lead to concern, they often need to know more in order to fulfill the law (Institute to Transform Child Protection, 2025). Getting more information does not require educators to conduct an investigation. Rather, it can be as simple as asking open-ended questions of students, such as "I heard you say that you did not eat dinner last night. Can you tell me more about that?" It can also sound like reaching out directly to families: "Your child arrived to class smelling like marijuana today. I wanted to connect with you because I'm concerned. I'd really like to hear from you about this. And before we get started, I want to remind you that I'm a mandatory reporter. So, if I have information about something that immediately and directly challenges a child's safety, I must share that information with appropriate authorities. I'm not sure that's necessary—I really want to start by talking with you."

A more intensive family engagement strategy, evidence-based home visiting, can cut maltreatment in half (Doe, Osborne, Huffman, Craig, & Shero, 2024; Levey, et al., 2017; van der Put, Assink, Gubbels, & van Solinge, 2021). The most effective programs focus on family strengths, assume that adults in the lives of the child are equal partners and connect families to aid for specific challenges (MacLeod & Nelson, 2000; Venkateswaran, Laird, Robles, & Jeffries, 2018). Evaluations of the national Parent Teacher Home Visit project show that visiting 10 percent of students is linked to schoolwide improvements in attendance and academic proficiency, as well as stronger family engagement, with both educators and parents thinking differently about each other (Sheldon & Jung, 2018; McKnight, Venkateswaran, Laird, Robles, & Shalev, 2017).

Wraparound the whole family: Sometimes, escalating interventions are necessary to address rising concerns. Responsive support to families is the most effective way to prevent violence against children at home (Cuartas, et al., 2024). When faced with imminent concerns, trauma-informed educators rely on a collective approach to collaboratively identify and meet as many needs as possible (van der Put, Assink, Gubbels, & van Solinge, 2021). Work with colleagues to leverage the skills of relevant school partners, programs and staff who can help to meet specific needs, including professionals who work in counseling, family engagement, food service, nursing, psychology, social work, speech-language pathology and therapy. Conscientiously practice confidentiality through complex collaborations. Coordinating effective support does not require educators to be "trauma detectives" (Venet, 2021) Rather, focus on seeking and sharing actionable information.

Reflections

- How can you deepen relationships in your professional circle toward collaboration, curiosity, compassion and consultation?
- Review the "respond vs. react" framework (Itzkowitz & Olson, 2022). How many of the eight strategies briefly outlined to complement mandatory reporting are you confident in using?

Recommended resource

"Reimagining Mandated Reporting" by the Institute to Transform Child Protection, **vimeo.com/1072599814**

Healing centered engagement

This section introduces and contextualizes the work of Shawn Ginwright. His concept of healing centered engagement informs the whole book and especially the next several chapters, including "Show empathy," "Critically reflect," "Take loving political action" and "Foster imagination."

> *"I am more than what happened to me, I'm not just my trauma."*
>
> —Marcus, young Black man in a healing circle (Ginwright, 2018)

Trauma-informed care offers an important lens to support young people; it also has limitations. Sometimes, "trauma-informed care" focuses only on harm, injury and traumatic effects. Related programming can seem to say, "You are the worst thing that ever happened to you," a deficit-based message (Venet, 2021).

Trauma-informed educators use asset-driven strategies and understand that some traumatic events are collective. For example, populations that disproportionately suffer from natural and man-made disasters share a common experience. Furthermore, it is important to consider root causes and environmental contexts that cause collective harm. Simply treating individuals leaves toxic systems, policies and practices intact.

We cannot risk focusing on the treatment of traumatic effects rather than fostering possibility or well-being. The absence of disease doesn't constitute health. The absence of violence does not constitute peace. And the reduction of pathology—anxiety, anger, fear, sadness, distrust and triggers—doesn't constitute well-being—including hope, happiness, imagination and trust. Everyone wants to be happy, not just have less misery (Ginwright, 2018).

Healing centered engagement is grounded in political action, youth development and positive psychology. It requires curiosity about students' culture, autonomy, relationships, sense of meaning and aspirations (Ginwright, 2016; REX TV by YouthREX, 2021). Advancing student well-being also requires trauma-informed educators to grapple with discrimination and systemic oppression (Civitillo, Mayer, & Jugert, 2023).

Show empathy

Young people thrive when they fully leverage the capacity to create, sustain and grow healthy connections to others (Ginwright, 2018; National Scientific Council on the Developing Child, 2015). Trauma-informed educators who practice empathy open to the possibility of vulnerable and engaged presence to make emotional connections (Ham, 2024). They do not relinquish expectations or standards. Instead, they focus on removing obstacles to learning and modifying processes to increase chances of student success (Meyers, Rowell, Wells, & Smith, 2019).

Critically reflect

Seek student perspectives, reflect on your own perspective and reconcile differences in the two— to change, when needed, as well as to frame behaviors in a strengths-based way. A strong sense of self helps young people share experiences of community and belonging. Respect for culture includes attention to social identities that are constructed in the shadow of politicized differences, such as race, gender, (dis)ability status and sexual orientation (Ginwright, 2018).

Take loving political action

Young people need to exercise power and control in school. Trauma-informed educators help youth experience individual and collective action to both create and change the root causes of personal, social and community challenges (Gross, 2024). Young people also need to build awareness of justice and inequality and explore possibilities for their lives. Students heal when educators help them focus on their goals for personal and collective well-being, as well as how collective strengths can help achieve them.

Foster imagination

Trauma-informed educators guide young people's profound discoveries of who they are, where they are going and what purpose they were born to serve. Regularly engage young people in positive discussions about their futures. Social action contributes to overall well-being, hopefulness and optimism.

9 Show empathy

CONTENT NOTE. This chapter is not likely to upset or trigger readers with references to specific forms of harm.

> *"Our ability to learn relies on our brain's ability to change and adapt in response to a new experience through a diverse set of processes called neuroplasticity. In recent years scientists have discovered that the biological and genetic processes driving neuroplasticity are largely regulated by neural systems dedicated to emotional regulation, bonding, and attachment."*
>
> —Drulis, Matz, Samuelson and Cozolino (Restoring Relationships, Healing Trauma, and Creating Securely Attached Classrooms, 2021)

Young people thrive when they fully leverage the capacity to create, sustain and grow healthy connections to others (Ginwright, 2018). In fact, healthy relationships with adults are among the best ways to protect young people from harm and lasting traumatic effects (National Scientific Council on the Developing Child, 2015). Authentic, protective relationships are much more complicated than proximity. They require deliberate effort and emotional regulation, among other things. This chapter covers some of the key ingredients to showing empathy.

Elevate possibility over problems

The young brain is malleable or "plastic" (Wenger & Kühn, 2021). In other words, children's developing brains are quick to change. This makes children particularly susceptible to trauma; it also means that young people who receive whole child attention that addresses physical, social and environmental factors are typically incredibly resilient (Kopec & Harte, 2020). Despite serious adversity, many children can have positive outcomes, provided they have adequate support (National Scientific Council on the Developing Child, 2015).

Educators who work with students past the early childhood stage have incredible opportunities to contribute to student health and well-being. Neuroplasticity "makes adolescents particularly vulnerable to the impact of trauma. However, this period of development also offers the chance to heal from trauma experienced early in life when young people receive targeted support and intervention" (All4Ed, 2019). Research suggests that educators who work with elementary school age children may be most impactful with a focus on student confidence, competence and esteem, as well as the ability to reflect and take time to consider options when deciding to act, rather than behaving impulsively. For older students in middle and high school, research points trauma-informed educators toward encouraging a sense of personal responsibility related to an internalized set of values and socially perceptive and mature relationships (Blaustein & Kinniburgh, 2019).

Educators can build coping skills in the same way they support academic skill development: Scaffold for success. Guide reflection and connect specific skills to practice. Integrate expectations for coping and opportunities for practice into pre-assessments, self-reflections, activity instructions, rubrics and grading models.

Open to new connection

Sympathy, a pity-based response focused on preserving the observer, is not empathy. Empathy exists on a continuum. Empathy is not fixed, but plastic; it can change. It also requires effort: Empathy can be practiced and strengthened. Regularly practicing empathy is linked to students feeling more care from educators, as well as reduced reliance on social isolation (such as suspensions) for misbehavior (Meyers, Rowell, Wells, & Smith, 2019).

Practicing empathy means taking emotional risks by being more vulnerable, open and honest. Furthermore, modeling emotional literacy allows youth to examine their own complex feelings. For example, ask students to identify values that are important to them and then to explain why those values are important (Meyers, Rowell, Wells, & Smith, 2019).

Support to success

Trauma-informed educators who practice empathy do not lower standards or aspirations. They do not withhold valuable instruction. Rather, they see students' capacity and potential and focus on removing obstacles to learning and modifying processes to increase chances of student success (Meyers, Rowell, Wells, & Smith, 2019; Venet, 2021). High levels of support are tailored to address the specific student's strengths, abilities, background, skills, culture and/or preferences, and to help students meet high expectations (Venet, 2021; Kieran & Anderson, 2019).

A trauma-informed educator also prioritizes (re)designing environments for inclusion over making accommodations that depend on student disclosure, diagnosis or labeling (Kopec & Harte, 2020). Research supports using the following ABCs of empathy, environmental shifts, and process changes to help students achieve objectives (Meyers, Rowell, Wells, & Smith, 2019; Warren, 2014).

ABCs of Empathy

- **Address** the whole child.
- **Build** flexibility into due dates.
- **Create** transparent assignments.
    - » Identify purpose and learning objectives.
    - » Provide instructions for steps to take.
    - » Provide clear criteria for success.
- **Design** course policies to reflect a deep understanding of social situations.
    - » Provide opportunities to redo/retake.
    - » Use flexibility "tokens"—all students receive set number and types of flexibility in a given period (e.g., retake, redo, submit late) with no questions asked. Explain boundaries in advance (e.g., may not be used on group projects, cannot be used after final grades are submitted to administrators).
- **Explain** the rationale behind classroom rules or policies; this may be easily achieved by developing classroom norms with students and eliciting their reasoning.
- **Flexibly consider** student difference.
- **Get** to know students.
- **Hold** students in high esteem while practicing curiosity about outcomes.
- **Invite** students to openly express their values and priorities.
    - » Listen intently.
    - » Ask clarifying questions.
    - » Demonstrate attentiveness.
    - » Share gratitude or advice in response.
- **Know** the neighborhood(s) surrounding the school and students' families.
- **Leverage** prior knowledge of students' cultures; learn more.
- **Make** yourself available for inquiry.
- **Organize** and structure time for student expression.

- **Prioritize** student learning; accommodations do not become "opt-outs."
- **Review** the possible role of adversity and systemic oppression.
- **Support** effective time management with explicit ideas and instructions.
- **Take** an asset-based approach.
- **Utilize** the language of "family."

Reflections

Share a routine that helps you understand students' context or circumstances.

- What are the steps?
- When do you typically use this routine?
- What are the time parameters for this routine?
- How does this routine ensure high standards for students?

Recommended resource

"The Future of Healing: Shifting From Trauma Informed Care to Healing Centered Engagement" by Shawn Ginwright, **medium.com/@ginwright/the-future-of-healing-shifting-from-trauma-informed-care-to-healing-centered-engagement-634f557ce69c**

10 Critically reflect

CONTENT NOTE. This chapter includes ideas related to systemic oppression.

> *"There cannot be caring without justice, and justice without caring."*
>
> —Virginia Held (The Ethics of Care: Personal, Political, and Global, 2005)

In addition to showing empathy, trauma-informed educators consider students' sociopolitical context—including historical, cultural, ethnic, economic and other systemic circumstances that deeply influence their identities. This chapter covers some big picture ideas and concepts to inform active engagement and conversation with students about systems that impact their opportunities, outcomes and worldview.

Analyze the conditions of traumatic environments

In the U.S., social identities are formed based on things like ability, age, class, ethnicity, height, language skills, legal and migration status, race, religion, sexuality and weight. In every society, people choose which identity markers will be ascribed social meaning. For example, there are significant disparities in career trajectories for tall people, compared to short ones. As another example, differences in income and class status are linked to significantly different health and quality of life outcomes. While individuals do not always fit the broader group patterns, comparisons across groups based on these markers reveal that social identity influences access to power, prestige, acceptability and validity, opportunity, expectations, punishment, leisure, time, capital and representation.

These patterns are present and pervasive. Yet we cannot make the mistake of thinking that systemic oppression is natural or rational. These social outcomes are not inherent (Wallis, 2020; Marya & Patel, 2021). People also differ by eyelash length, shoe size, preferred leisure activities and other characteristics. But we don't use any of those to organize our social identities or social outcomes. Rather, we—as a collective—design, accept and perpetuate inequitable distribution of resources and related dignity. Systemic oppression names this historic and persistent inequity, as well as how we arrive here.

Levers of oppression

The following framework is grounded in the work of literacy teacher and political philosopher, Paolo Friere (Pedagogy of the Oppressed, 2007) and adapted from multiple sources (Shlasko, 2015; Roberts, 2022; Trent, Dooley, & Douge, 2019; Mayes, 2022). We offer one way to think about systemic oppression and *how* these sociocultural patterns come to exist (Shlasko, 2015; Ginwright, 2016):

- **Violence** includes physical, sexual and emotional violence; the threat of violence; and policies and structures that normalize and condone violence.
- **Culture of Silence** is a pattern of normalizing other levers of oppression by denying or minimizing their existence and impacts, as well as a pattern of rationalizing and reinforcing inequity as divine, inherent, unavoidable or natural.
- **Powerlessness** is a pattern of deprivation of the ability to make decisions about one's living or working conditions.
- **Cultural Imperialism** is the valuing and enforcement of a preferred or dominant group's culture, norms and characteristics.
- **Marginalization** is the prevention or limitation of full participation in society through exclusion from things like the job market, housing and geographic communities, health care system, public benefits programs or community activities.
- **Exploitation** is the systematic transfer of resources—such as land, wealth or labor value—from one group to another.
- **Policing** is the selective application of social expectations and legal rules to enforce and normalize other levers of oppression. Policing tactics are not limited to people with jobs in law enforcement and include coercion, confinement, control, corralling, detention, displacement, eviction, harassment, incarceration, intimidation and surveillance.

Effects of oppression

Like more acute or "obvious" forms of adversity, such as witnessing domestic violence or the death of a parent, systemic oppression seriously threatens health and well-being. People in systemically targeted groups face elevated risks of toxic stress and traumatic effects because they face chronic, traumatic exposure to oppression. Repeated exposure to systemic oppression can foster significant challenges, including (Ungar, 2013; Gilligan, 2011; DeAngelis, 2019; Kiss, et al., 2022; Hall, 2018; Trent, Dooley, & Douge, 2019; Táíwò, Fehrenbacher, & Cooke, 2021; Link & Phelan, 1995; Forde, Crookes, Suglia, & Demmer, 2019; Marya & Patel, 2021):

- Accelerated aging and early onset of health challenges
- Anger
- Avoidance, withdrawal, mistrust and reluctance to interact with people in the preferred or dominant group
- Grief and bereavement
- Hypervigilance to threat
- Irritability
- Lack of hopefulness for the future
- Low self-esteem
- Mental health challenges, including clinical anxiety and depression
- Poor concentration and distractibility
- Reduced access to resources for well-being, including capital, health services and employment
- Shame and humiliation
- Substance misuse and abuse

Further, acute violence exposure intersects with systemic oppression for disproportionate impact on marginalized children (Bor, Venkataramani, Williams, & Tsai, 2018). For example, "witnessing racism due to coronavirus" was among the top predictive factors for depressive symptoms among adolescents during the pandemic (Kiss, et al., 2022). Systemic oppression is also linked to serious implications for learning, including fear of failure, stereotype threat and feeling uncertain about belonging (Meyers, Rowell, Wells, & Smith, 2019). Finally, overall systemic oppression produces and exploits group-differentiated vulnerability to premature death (Gilmore, 2022). Systemic oppression is linked to traumatic effects that can carry into future generations, which is linked to problems in school even decades after the initial traumatic exposure (DeAngelis, 2019; Newland, 2022).

Reflections

Adverse Childhood Experiences (ACE) Study: An Overview

Starting in 1995, the U.S. Centers for Disease Control and Prevention (CDC) and Kaiser Permanente conducted one of the largest studies on childhood adversity and its impacts into adulthood. The Adverse Childhood Experiences (ACE) study examined the following traumatic events and exposures:

- Emotional, physical and sexual abuse
- Domestic violence
- Substance abuse
- Mental illness
- Parental separation or divorce
- Incarceration of a household member
- Emotional and physical neglect

The study linked increased adverse exposure to elevated risk for poor health and quality of life, including increased likelihood for injury, mental illness, maternal health challenges, infectious disease, chronic disease and reduced opportunities for economic mobility (U.S. Centers for Disease Control and Prevention, 2021).

- The initial ACE study did not explore racism, sexism, homophobia or other systemic oppression as possible sources of trauma. Compare and contrast the possible effects of systemic oppression with the list of ACE impacts above. What would you expect might be the impacts of the initial, limited definition of ACEs?
- What has best prepared you to interrupt systemic oppression as a pervasive traumatic exposure?

Recommended resource

Equity-Centered Trauma-Informed Education by Alex Shevrin Venet

11 Take loving political action

CONTENT NOTE. This chapter includes ideas related to civil disobedience, racism, shame and slavery.

> *"Youth organizing has different goals than school. They're about building young people's power and capacity and voice. That's what organizing is for. That's not what school is for, right? School is for trying to trick kids into forgetting that they have any power."*
>
> —Carla Shalaby (Cooper & Thesing, 2023)

When harm is political, healing must be, as well. Trauma-informed educators embrace organizing as political healing (Venet, 2021; Ginwright, 2018; Gross, 2024). When done well, organizing for, and participating in, collective action can be healing whether it leads to a win—because it affirms the agency, dignity and strengths of those engaged.

Get uncomfortable

Loving political action directly challenges some people's comfort to achieve greater safety and well-being for all, with special attention to increased safety for marginalized people. Ginwright defines loving political action as student-led collective action (2018). Venet adds that educators must also practice solidarity and social justice efforts to make collective action impactful (2021). By elevating social duties to each other, as equal members of a school community trauma-informed educators work to build learning communities of "shared sacrifice, shared risk, shared reward" (Hunt-Hendrix & Taylor, 2024).

Union organizing can be a powerful tool to reduce the risk and discomfort of collective action and solidarity. Importantly, the National Labor Relations Act protects "concerted activity" by workers, including circulating a petition and joining with colleagues to speak with decision-makers directly about problems (National Labor Relations Board).

An Example of Protected Concerted Activity

In 2016, a group called Social Equity Educators wanted to conduct a citywide activity in support of Black students' lives. But they worried that some colleagues would participate in a visibility action with T-shirts and others would opt out. They were concerned that educators who did not participate could send the wrong message. They considered that some educators might be threatened or face retaliation. To move forward, they approached their union with a brief resolution calling on all educators in the district to join a day of action, a resolution that easily passed (Au & Hagopian, 2018).

Interrupt shame

Guilt is the feeling that one has done something wrong; shame is the feeling that a mistake reveals that oneself is inherently wrong. Shame is a powerful social emotion. Systemic oppression can be internalized by the oppressed as shameful—as evidence that a socially sidelined trait is proof that one is indeed less than human.

Clint Smith, a former teacher and Black historian, offers an example of counteracting shame. Here, he clarifies a perspective shift that helped him to better understand and align with his enslaved ancestors:

> *"I was angered by the stories of those who did not escape. Had they not tried hard enough? Didn't they care enough to do something? Did they choose to remain enslaved? This, I now realize, is part of the insidiousness of white supremacy. It illuminates the exceptional in order to implicitly blame those who cannot, despite the most brutal circumstances, attain superhuman heights. It does this instead of blaming the system, the people who built it, and the people who maintained it."*
> *—Clint Smith (How the Word is Passed, 2022)*

Smith models key steps to effectively disrupt shame. First, he engages in multiple open, structured dialogues in his book, *How the Word Is Passed: A Reckoning with the History of Slavery Across America*—and provides a condensed version of his realizations in the quote as he works to identify with the oppressed. Second, he recognizes how deficit thinking framed his previous approach to historical content, such as by remembering that he has asked, "Had they not tried hard enough?" Finally, he redirects and attends to power. Other educators have worked to interrupt shame by naming that they love people who have been incarcerated (Sokolower, 2018) and by tracing trauma in their family tree to move beyond secrets (DeAngelis, 2019).

Share power in student-led community problem-solving

Modern education should prepare students to transform the social conditions of their oppression (Táíwò O. , 2022). Trauma-informed educators learn alongside students in pursuit of a just world. There are several ways to think about integrating healing justice into work with students.

Project-based learning to challenge oppression

Dismantling and challenging the root causes of systemic oppression is essential to healing (Ginwright, 2018). Trauma-informed educators are creative in applying this concept with students, from assigning documentaries and partnering with universities on action research with middle school students (Venet, 2021) to researching how many U.S. presidents were slave owners with elementary school students, role playing as grassroots civil rights activists in high school and more (Watson, Hagopian, & Au, 2018). Fundamentally, trauma-informed educators affirm students' ideas as valuable.

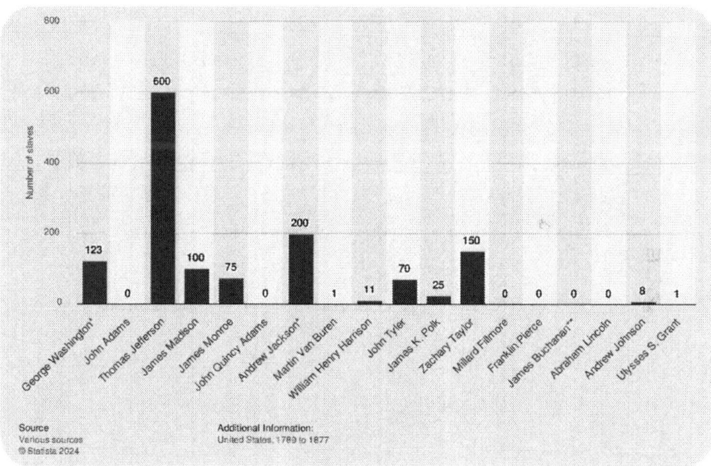

Reported number of slaves owned by U.S. presidents who served from 1789 to 1877 (Statista, 2020).

*Number of slaves owned at time of death. Washington personally owned 123 slaves, although there were as many as 317 working on his property at the time of his death.
**Buchanan is believed to have bought slaves, whom he immediately freed and employed as servants.

Resistance as cultural legacy

Students benefit from knowing the ways their communities have used political strategies to achieve radical new ends. Resistance to systemic oppression often engenders unique resilience strategies that may appear as cultural legacies (Whitbeck, Adams, Hoyt, & Chen, 2004), such as:

- Specific traditions, practices and rituals
- Histories of resistance and the ways communities have strategized for change
- Culturally specific coping and healing approaches
- Messaging, art and archives that directly combat shame related to identity

For example, scholars recognize diverse resilience practices—including place attachment, collective history and economies structured around gifts—as essential to the ongoing tenacity of Indigenous people of the Americas (Ford, et al., 2020; Kirmayer, Dandeneau, Marshall, Phillips, & Williamson, 2011; Kimmerer, 2015). As another example, pride in and strong connection to Blackness are protective against white supremacy and anti-Black racism (Wallis, 2020). Trauma-informed educators seek to partner with families to learn more about their specific approaches to coping and resilience, in order to guide and participate in strategies for healing that may best resonate with students.

Intentional presence

Not every moment with students will be filled with complex explorations of power; some will be about listening, sharing and being wholly alive with each other. Even everyday interactions should carry the "Four Rs" of respect, responsibility, relationality and reciprocity (Petrone & Rogers Stanton, 2021). Overall, a trauma-informed educator's work with students must be aimed toward transformational, hopeful and constructive solutions (Venet, 2021).

Reflections

- What is the role of a trauma-informed educator in supporting student-led political action?
- Where in your daily routines are there opportunities for student-led political action?

Recommended resource

Teaching for Black Lives edited by Dyan Watson, Jessie Hagopian and Wayne Au

12 Foster imagination

CONTENT NOTE. This chapter includes ideas related to the following: anxiety, depression, illness, mental health issues and suicide.

> *"Young children learn best by acting out the world around them, by putting themselves in other people's shoes. We can repeat the narratives of the powerful, or we can give students the chance to see the world through the eyes of the people who are most vulnerable, and those who are trying to work for justice."*
>
> —Editors of Rethinking Schools (Little Kids, Big Ideas: Teaching Social Issues and Global Conflicts with Young Children, 2019)

When he first published, Ginwright included core suggestions to help educators make his ideas about healing centered engagement come to fruition in work with students: Show empathy, build critical reflection, take loving political action and foster imagination. This last recommendation included the call to create activities and opportunities for young people to play, reimagine, design and envision their lives (Ginwright, 2018). In this chapter, we focus on the power and complexity of play to developing minds.

The value of play

Play is linked to lower levels of the stress hormone, cortisol. Play increases the brain's plasticity, or openness to change. Play can enhance curiosity, which facilitates memory and learning (Yogman, Garner, Hutchinson, Hirsh-Pasek, & Golinkoff, 2018). Playing at school boosts kids' physical fitness, attentiveness, cognition and social skills (Ramstetter & Murray, 2017). But over the last 70 years, children have been playing less (Gray, Lancy, & Bjorklund, 2023).

The U.S. has significantly changed the way we talk about children. We have stopped assuming they are competent, responsible and resilient; instead, we stress their need for protection and monitoring. And we have filled their lives with supervision.

Between 1981 and 2003, the average amount of time that early elementary students spent on homework and school increased by

11.4 hours

per week

(Gray, Lancy, & Bjorklund, 2023).

Children exhibit less independence, such as walking to school, biking or riding buses. They spend more time in school, with the average academic year covering five more weeks than it did in 1950. Kids today have less access to recess than previous generations. And on average, children's time in school and on homework total more than 50 hours per week, making academic expectations more rigorous than the 40-hour work week (Gray, Lancy, & Bjorklund, 2023).

During the same 70-year span, children's mental health has declined. Depression, anxiety, sadness, hopelessness and youth suicide have all increased. School may be part of the problem: At the start of the 21st century, recess access began to decline as pressures to prepare for high-stakes testing increased (Ramstetter & Murray, 2017). Students are twice as likely to go to the emergency room, attempt and complete suicide during a week they have school as during a week they are scheduled to be on vacation (Gray, Lancy, & Bjorklund, 2023).

School can also be part of the solution: Adding recess boosts emotional well-being and has at least a neutral effect on academic gains. Assignments like the "Let Grow" project, which encourages students to go home and do something that they have never done before, *without an adult*, impact both students' self-perception and parents' ideas of kids' competence (Stand Together, 2023).

Leverage play at school

Borrow from the building blocks of play to strengthen learning and well-being (Gray P., 2017):

- **Autonomy:** Play is directed by the players (not by adults); encourage student autonomy and authentic control or choice.
- **Belonging:** Young people receive social support, as needed, with natural back-and-forth interactions that require them to share, negotiate and problem-solve.
- **Competence:** Players have sufficient skill to pursue freely chosen paths without monitoring or supervision.
- **Discovery:** Play includes taking risks, experimenting and testing boundaries, yet is typically buffered from real-life consequences.
- **Engagement:** Children develop skills that are useful to themselves and their communities.

Trauma-informed educators proactively integrate play by considering which types of play best align with students' developmental stage (Blaustein & Kinniburgh, 2019; Yogman, Garner, Hutchinson, Hirsh-Pasek, & Golinkoff, 2018).

- Young children tend to enjoy imaginary play (e.g., playing nurse or truck driver), reading and telling stories, complex motor tasks (balancing on a beam, jumping rope, climbing, riding a bike) and cooperative board games to achieve a goal as a team.
- Elementary school students tend to be more interested in interactive game play, rules/boundaries and strategy. They tend to enjoy board games that require planning (e.g., chess, checkers), memory, logic and reasoning games, movement games that require concentration (e.g., Red Light, Green Light) and music-based play (e.g., singing, dancing and playing an instrument).
- Adolescents tend to enjoy complex play, such as sports, drama and art. These activities allow older students to authentically use rapidly developing executive skills, including self-monitoring, goal setting, organization, planning and socializing.

Especially with younger students, trauma-informed educators practice deliberately communicating emotional literacy as part of play activities, such as by narrating a student's behavior out loud and discussing emotions as they play.

Play is political, too

"For the most part, schools value quiet children over loud ones and operate as though adults are the only teachers in the room. The adults get to speak while the young people listen. Questions are answered rather than asked. Our schools are designed to prepare children to take their assumed place in the social order rather than to question and challenge that order. Because we train youth in the image of capitalism instead of a vision of freedom—for lives as individual workers rather than solitary human beings—young people are taught academic content that can be drilled and tested rather than understanding literacies and numeracies as forms of power, tools for organizing, fodder of the development of their own original ideas."
—Carla Shalaby (Troublemakers: Lessons in Freedom from Young Children at School, 2017)

Play can be boisterous—and some children are more likely than others to be monitored for being "too loud" or seemingly "out of control." Play can be imitative—and some students are more likely than others to be punished for appearing "adult-like." Play can provide counterbalance to serious and necessary activities—and some people are more likely than others to be seen as deserving of leisure (Trey, 2025; McPherson, 2021; Ramstetter & Murray, 2017). Unsupervised play can be liberatory and capacity-building—and some children's families are more likely than others to be accused of neglect if their kids play alone (Itzkowitz & Olson, 2022).

Modeling and role-playing can help students of all developmental stages to focus on resolving realistic conflicts (Wright, 2017). Moreover, games that challenge players to practice empathy activate a shared sense of humanity and can provide a basis for dialogue on more complex concepts, such as power and systems of oppression (Boltz, Henriksen, Mishra, & Deep-Play Research Group, 2015). Role play can also be misused, so trauma-informed educators carefully consider "whose voices we privilege, whose stories we put center stage" (Editors of Rethinking Schools, 2019).

Reflections

- How is play related to toxic stress and trauma?
- How is the decrease in play time during the school day affecting students socially and academically?

Recommended resource

"Time to Play: Recognizing the Benefits of Recess" by Catherine Ramstetter and Robert Murray, **aft.org/ae/spring2017**

Regulate, relate, reason

This section introduces Bruce Perry's Neurosequential Model of Therapeutics (NMT), which challenges trauma-informed educators to appreciate when "talking it out" is appropriate—and when it is not—with attention to the way the brain develops. His research informs the entire course and especially the next few chapters, including "Prevent re-traumatization," "Teach diverse coping skills," "Facilitate positive experiences" and "De-escalate stressful scenarios."

Trauma-informed educators proactively prevent harm and toxic stress by establishing routines and environments that help students experience and expect safety, certainty and (self-) control. Conflicts and tension still emerge and then NMT becomes essential (Perry, 2020). The model is grounded in an understanding of how brains have changed over thousands of years.

The brain stem evolved first and is associated with basic survival, such as breathing, balance or equilibrium, maintaining a functional temperature and eating. The middle brain is associated with more complex demands, including making meaning of diverse stimuli and emotions. The cortex, or frontal lobes, are most recently evolved and most closely related to learning, including producing and parsing language, imagining and orienting around alternative perspectives and problem solving. Being extremely upset or having an acute trauma response impacts every part of the brain. Perry advocates three general steps to help students reset and return to learning, each aligned with one general section of the brain. Importantly, he insists that interventions start simple and become more complex, following the brain's organization.

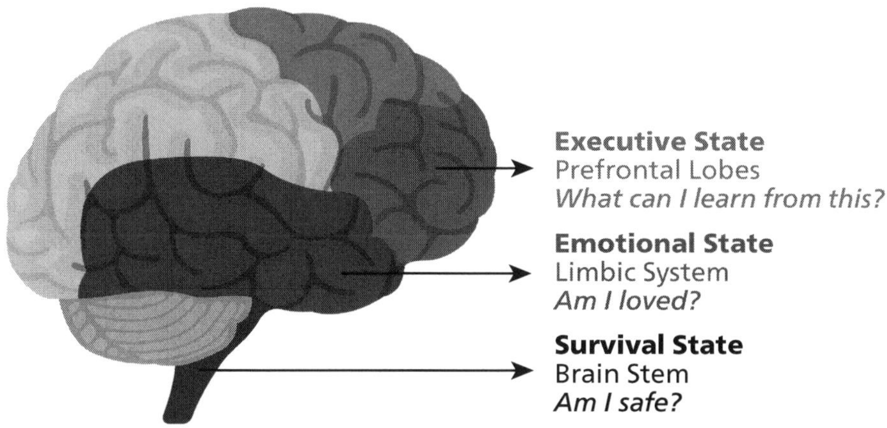

The Neurosequential Model of Therapeutics encourages educators to address the demands of the stressed or escalated child by following the brain in a 'bottom up' approach. First, address safety with regulation, then (re)establish connection with relational strategies and finally, integrate new concepts with reasoning.

Regulate: Escalated students, and especially those experiencing peak distress, are primarily operating from the brain stem and a survival state. They are having a severe stress response and focused on coping to survive. At this stage, the student may seem inconsolable; emotional literacy, reteaching coping skills and repeating rules or expectations are ineffective. More input—even well-meaning ideas like, "Calm down" and "Take deep breaths"—is overwhelming. Indeed, trying to "talk it out" can be inflammatory and lead to more problems. To help a student de-escalate when accelerated or in peak distress, prioritize brain stem regulation (Public School Notebook, 2018; Perry, 2020):

- Disengage and decrease stimuli while the student is in a safe space to allow them to regain some composure.
- Leverage existing resources and strategies the student has already mastered; do not try to introduce or reinforce anything new.
- Project safety and calm assertively and without words, such as through open posture and soft eye contact.
- Minimize stimuli, including unnecessary words or physical contact. Increase the escalated student's personal space.
- Encourage access to a safe, warm and comforting space, if available. Warm blankets, plushies and large pillows can make for inviting spaces; clay, playdoh, "fidgets" and spinners can be helpful, as well.
- Encourage safe, full body movement, such as stomping, walking to another space or moving something substantial like a backpack, to ground and engage large muscles (arms, legs and torso). Bilateral (side to side) and rhythmic physical activity are also effective; these may include stimming, rocking in a chair or bouncing on a ball.

For students recovering from acceleration or peak distress, use independent work, reduced social demands and minimal adult engagement. Social isolation is not necessarily helpful for students learning to reintegrate into the community following an episode of peak distress. Physical regulation—including steady breathing, smooth movements and easy balance—is a good sign that students are ready to de-escalate their middle brain and deal with emotions.

Relate: Whether in recovery or agitation, students may feel afraid of their own lack of control, guilty that they mishandled escalation or a trigger, shame at their stress response or other emotions, in addition to their feelings about the initial challenge. To best support students who need to relate:

- Listen and repeat student ideas without judgment.
- Acknowledge and name emotions; name and observe behaviors.
- Offer encouragement, reassurance and a sense of belonging.

- Practice empathy.
- Share power in your posture, such as by sitting side-by-side.

De-escalate an agitated student by using brief distractions, such as by asking for help with a classroom errand or special project. Once a student is ready to be engaged—such as by exchanging eye contact and attempting to name or process feelings—they are likely ready to move to the final stage in NMT: reasoning.

Reason: Only after the previous stages are resolved, revisit the incident or challenge. Before and during a student encounter focused on rules, expectations, strategies or planning, check for indicators that they are calm and engaged—that their brains are ready for the complex thinking ahead.

- Together, identify the problem, as well as possible triggers.
- Guide problem-solving, such as through coaching, role play, mentorship or thinking about multiple scenarios, pathways and outcomes.
- Clearly distinguish between disapproval of choices and behaviors from disappointment in a person to avoid shame.

13 Prevent re-traumatization

CONTENT NOTE. This chapter includes ideas related to specific trauma triggers.

> *"When asked how they define school safety, the girls and young women emphasized the emotional and psychological aspects of safety. They expressed that feeling safe includes the following: feeling comfortable; not having to worry; not being afraid of getting hurt or needing to watch one's back; being able to express oneself and have safe spaces to exist within; having supportive, nonjudgmental adults around; and having mental health and emotional support in schools."*
>
> —Bernadel, et al. (Keep Her Safe: Centering Black Girls in School Safety, 2024)

Trauma triggers make a past traumatic event feel real here and now, often instigating a new trauma response and exacerbating existing traumatic effects. This chapter focuses on how trauma-informed educators can work to both prevent triggering traumatized students and hold meaningful lines between the past and present.

Trauma triggers

A trigger is an antecedent or a catalyst. Lots of behaviors and responses have triggers—they can take the form of sight, sound, touch, smell or taste (Dombo & Sabatino, 2019). For example, children's whining often triggers adult annoyance. And young people's tiredness, hunger and boredom often catalyze their acting out (Day, et al., 2017). But a trauma trigger is not "just like" any other trigger. It's the result of an altered stress response (Wilson, Hansen, & Li, 2011).

Trauma triggers act as sudden reminders and set off repeat trauma responses. The child relives a loss of power, control or safety and activates survival strategies as if the initial event is happening again in the present moment (Tippett, 2015; Substance Abuse and Mental Health Services Administration, 2014). This re-traumatization continues to demand emergency-oriented brain functions, bodily responses and behaviors—and fundamentally inhibits learning. It can also lead to aggression, anger and withdrawal. Re-traumatization interrupts others' learning, too (Day, et al., 2017; Dombo & Sabatino, 2019).

Because traumatic memories are relived more than recalled, students may not be clear about why a trigger bothers them and may not even be aware of a pattern in their responses to triggers (Tippett, 2015). Trauma-informed educators practice curiosity and connection when they observe an acute trauma response. Consider additional information the student can share that may help in recognizing a trigger (Dombo & Sabatino, 2019):

- How do they express distress?
- What does the student seek to (re)establish safety?
- What in the environment suggested the loss of safety?
- What helps the student consent to be vulnerable? In other words, what works to show that you are a person who can support their survival and their thriving?

Mitigate and minimize environmental triggers

By deliberately managing students' potential trauma triggers (and our own behavioral triggers), we are not *treating* traumatic effects. We are not trying to protect students from their emotions or eliminate all stressors. Rather, we are trying to help students learn effective ways to calm their brain and body and practice resilience: to notice, reduce and work through challenges (Cooper & Thesing, 2023). Addressing triggers can include efforts to (Cummings, Addante, Swindell, & Meadan, 2017; Venet, 2021; Prax & O'Connor, 2018):

- Acknowledge transitions (announce in advance where possible), such as between activities and between major shifts in the week.
- Acknowledge jarring sounds (announce in advance where possible), such as alarms during drills, bells that accompany schedule changes and regular loudspeaker activation.
- Correct or comment on undesirable student behavior out of the public eye.
- Model seeking and giving enthusiastic consent for physical contact.
- Muffle and reduce noise with rugs and noise-absorbing fabrics.
- Seat students to encourage equitable contributions (e.g., in a circle instead of rows).
- Strategically place adult support during drills, such as to assist with emergency vehicles and personnel, as well as loud sounds and changes in routine.
- Use lamps or cover overhead fluorescent lights.
- Use door stops to prevent slamming; replace doors with covered windows or screens.

Constructive environments

A traumatic experience is physically and psychologically threatening. Trauma-informed learning environments therefore elevate both physical and psychological safety, such as by reducing chaos and by extending meaningful power, control and choice to students (Dombo & Sabatino, 2019).

Practicing empathy and facilitating positive social experiences are critical to building these learning environments. Furthermore, even after dramatic and atypical trauma exposure, students crave engaging, focused and challenging learning opportunities with warm and responsive educators (Day, et al., 2017).

Structure and routines, follow-through with logical plans and calm demeanor—even when stressed—are also essential ingredients to trauma-informed learning environments. These planning and self-regulation skills modeled by educators help students successfully regulate their own emotions and behavior, effectively de-escalate when necessary, strengthen protective relationships and ultimately learn (Guarino & Chagnon, 2018; Prax & O'Connor, 2018).

Reflections

- Which trauma triggers are most relevant or common to your student population?
- Which trauma triggers are most influenced by your administration or other layers of power beyond your direct control?

Recommended resource

"Trauma Care in Schools" by Eileen Dombo and Christine Sabatino, **aft.org/ae/summer2019/dombo_sabatino**

14 Teach diverse coping skills

CONTENT NOTE. This chapter is not likely to upset or trigger readers with references to specific forms of harm.

> *"Although we were flawed, we were marvelous, too."*
> —Daniel Black (Don't Cry For Me, 2022)

Trauma-informed educators construct calm and consistent learning environments. To further prevent re-traumatization, they also help students build resilience, practice effective coping and regulate their physical and emotional responses when upset.

Adapting to stress

Wherever researchers study risk and adversity, they also find coping and resilience, or "successful adaptation despite challenging or threatening circumstances" (Blaustein & Kinniburgh, 2019). Resilience is the result of protective circumstances and a skill set that grounds hopefulness, such as learning who to ask, when to ask and how to ask for help. Every child is resilient and has adapted to survive in her world. But survival strategies are not always aligned with thriving. Positive experiences and protective factors "tilt" a child's life in a positive direction. Loving and supportive relationships with healthy adults are especially protective and can prevent the stress response from becoming toxic (Centers for Disease Control and Prevention, 2018; Yule, Houston, & Grych, 2019). Indeed, we want students to adapt skills and strategies for more than surviving danger or weathering deprivation; we want to "tip" them toward well-being. To help students establish complex resilience skills, trauma-informed educators need to understand how students develop coping capacity.

Developing resilience

Very early in life, many children learn to express feelings, soothe themselves and react to others' emotions. Children generally establish more coping skills as they face increasing distress; as children grow, so does their ability to regulate their emotions and stress. The most effective individual protective factor for children is self-regulation. While coping is often shaped by temperament, it can also be learned (Liu, et al., 2020; Yule, Houston, & Grych, 2019). Trauma-informed educators focus on helping young people strengthen resilience at each developmental stage, such as through role play (Zimmer-Gembeck & Skinner, 2016; Blaustein & Kinniburgh, 2019; Yule, Houston, & Grych, 2019):

- **Infancy.** Adhere to sleep and meal routines; express and accept affection and positive temperament.
- **Preschool.** Seek and ask for support; tolerate being upset; provide themselves age-appropriate structure; increase independence.
- **Middle childhood.** Experience mastery and confidence; express positive self-esteem; reflect rather than react impulsively; use multiple skills, including humor, to cope when upset; participate in positive peer and adult relationships.
- **Adolescence.** Show personal responsibility and social maturity; demonstrate a belief in control over their outcomes and a desire to act purposefully; set and independently move toward goals; establish and act on personal values.

Coping strategies are contextual

Effective coping protects young people from developing traumatic effects. To determine which coping approaches are the most effective, researchers tend to group coping strategies and then compare outcomes between children who use one with children who tend to use another. One common contrast is between engaged or active coping (which includes problem-solving, thinking differently about the problem, seeking information or support and taking concrete action) with avoidant coping (which includes distraction, ignoring, denial, minimization, self-blame and self-criticism, resigned acceptance, venting, social withdrawal, escape and wishful thinking). Generally, avoidant coping is associated with higher levels of distress and illness (Bistricky, et al., 2019; Schibalski, et al., 2017). Active coping is especially adaptive when young people reasonably expect to exercise control, such as at school. While avoidant and emotion-based coping are overall linked to increased stress, in situations where students do not have much (or any) control over stressor(s), these coping approaches can also help young people adapt and adjust (Zimmer-Gembeck & Skinner, 2016).

Researchers have also compared coping approaches that focus on managing emotional reactions to challenges with coping that focuses on solving problems. Emotion-based coping is more predictive of health challenges, such as clinical depression and anxiety, than problem-solving (Zimmer-Gembeck & Skinner, 2016).

Having more strategies does not always mean more *effective* strategies. Students benefit from the assistance of trauma-informed educators to identify, adapt and evaluate approaches to fit the situation or challenge. However, helping students to deal with adversity does not absolve caring adults from the responsibility to genuinely endeavor to eliminate the root causes of harm. Changing circumstances and the demands of the learning environment often require more from adults than of children (Ellis, et al., 2020). In other words, boosting students' coping capacity is a complement, not a replacement, for a trauma-informed educators' robust work.

Reflections

- What kinds of redirection or coaching can you use to encourage students to move away from, or appropriately contextualize, maladaptive coping strategies?
- How is regulation related to liberation and healing?

Recommended resource

"Hidden Talents in Harsh Environments" by Bruce Ellis, Laura Abrams, Ann Masten, Robert Sternberg, Nim Tottenham and Willem Frankenhuis, **researchgate.net/profile/Bruce-Ellis-5/publication/342989483_Hidden_talents_in_harsh_environments/links/5f13aaa14585151299a6e691/Hidden-talents-in-harsh-environments.pdf**

15 Facilitate positive experiences

CONTENT NOTE. This chapter is not likely to upset or trigger readers with references to specific forms of harm.

> *"When you have resilience, you harness inner strength that helps you rebound from a setback or challenge, such as a job loss, an illness, a disaster or the death of a loved one. If you lack resilience, you might dwell on problems, feel victimized, become overwhelmed or turn to unhealthy coping mechanisms, such as substance abuse. Resilience won't make your problems go away—but resilience can give you the ability to see past them, find enjoyment in life and better handle stress. If you aren't as resilient as you'd like to be, you can develop skills to become more resilient."*
>
> —Mayo Clinic (Souers & Hall, 2016)

Throughout the book, we've discussed the importance of protective factors to prevent traumatic events from becoming traumatic effects. This chapter is especially interested in the ways that educators' everyday practices can promote healing.

Protective factors

A combination of protective factors can enhance a child's ability to cope or bounce back from harmful traumatic effects, including: (Darling-Hammond, Flook, Cook-Harvey, Barron, & Osher, 2019; Yule, Houston, & Grych, 2019).

- Academic achievement and extended learning opportunities
- Appropriate interventions before, during and after challenges
- Cognitive skills such as problem-solving, responsible decision-making and perspective-taking
- Community that respects and celebrates students' identities and cultures
- Consistent practices and predictable routines
- Physical and emotional safety

- Physical and mental health
- Positive instructional strategies
- Relationships with caring and supportive adults
- Restorative behavior supports that teach skills such as taking responsibility and making amends
- Sense of agency ("I can make meaningful choices.")
- Sense of belonging, mastery and purpose
- Social and emotional competence
    - » **Self-awareness:** Identify emotions and accurate self-perceptions
    - » **Self-management:** Manage stress and feelings, control impulses and use diverse coping strategies
    - » **Social awareness:** Take others' perspectives, empathize and appreciate diversity
    - » **Relationship skills:** Communicate, help and cooperate for healthy relationships
    - » **Responsible decision-making:** Identify problems, evaluate, reflect and act with consideration for the well-being of oneself and others

Students' growth potential

Children's willingness to engage in learning is experience-dependent (Goldberg, 2022). In contexts with rich relational connections, emotional support and collaboration, students are more likely to de-escalate into the calm and concentration that ground strong, lasting learning. In contrast, in competitive, stressful, agitated environments, students are more likely to withdraw, become distracted and act out (Drulis, Matz, Samuelson, & Cozolino, 2021). Resilience is a skill set, an ability to adapt successfully—not a trait (Center on the Developing Child, 2015). Trauma-informed educators help students develop resilience and in turn, can attune brains, bodies and behaviors for healing (National Scientific Council on the Developing Child, 2015).

Healing gestures

Research strongly supports five regular practices that show young people love and care, operationalize protective factors and help students develop resilience (Futures Without Violence, 2024).

Listen: Encourage and model active and supportive listening. A positive school climate is one with norms that support respectful listening among all members of the community. Create processes that allow students to share and be heard. Remain curious and ask supportive questions.

Comfort: Create predictable routines and transitions for children so they know what to expect. Establish safe and cozy spaces where students can calm down when they are upset. Respond with kindness and compassion when a child is escalated or triggered. Use grounding techniques such as yoga, meditation, breathing games and affirmations to help students learn and practice emotional regulation, social awareness, self-awareness, relationship skills and anger management. Try playing music or ringing a meditation bell to signal that it's time to transition.

Collaborate: Plan for students to work together during in-school and after-school activities. Facilitate peers sharing strengths towards a common goal using agreed upon rules and expectations. Demonstrate to students that group work can help identify multiple solutions to problems and that some might be more effective than others. Teach problem-solving skills and encourage working through conflicts together. Teach nonviolent resolution skills and model a problem-solving process rather than just giving students answers. Notice when children are frustrated and offer supportive guidance. When possible, help them identify other sources of support in school, in the community and at home.

Inspire: Demonstrate a belief in your students' potential, create a climate of achievement by setting high standards and set a positive example as a role model through the ways you approach tasks and relationships. Help children identify their natural talents or abilities and use them in the classroom. Connect children to after-school programs such as theater, dance, sports and opportunities to join in community service. Create opportunities for children to learn about different career paths and take on leadership roles in and outside of the classroom. Explore their future goals and engage them in short and long-term goal setting—and establish realistic, achievable goals. Build community by inquiring about friend networks and helping students identify friends that make them feel happy and confident.

Celebrate: Recognize student efforts and encourage positive interactions between young people and their peers, as well as other educators. Engage children in open-ended, free play. Point out their talents and strengths and offer more opportunities to build on these skills, including with small wins and incremental progress. Publicly recognize and praise children when they are doing things right. When you need to re-direct their behavior, do it privately and calmly. Greet children by name and offer rounds of applause or high fives as encouragement. Take children's concerns seriously and offer validating statements. Tell them that you like them and why you think they're special.

Establish a climate of respect and ensure your interactions with students are affirming, encouraging and validating. Identify and reinforce a child's areas of strength and give positive reinforcement when they show skills like perseverance and focus. When children have setbacks or frustrations, praise their efforts and help them figure out next steps.

Reflection

- How can you help students understand that their brains are incredibly dynamic and changing (also called neuroplasticity)?
- Which recommendation in this chapter seems most aspirational or challenging for your school context? Which feels most attainable or easy to scale to more students, more often?

Recommended resource

"Supportive Relationships and Active Skill-Building Strengthen the Foundations of Resilience: Working Paper 13" by the National Scientific Council on the Developing Child, **developingchild.harvard.edu/resources/working-paper/supportive-relationships-and-active-skill-building-strengthen-the-foundations-of-resilience/**

16 De-escalate stressful scenarios

CONTENT NOTE. This chapter includes ideas related to trauma triggers.

> *"He used to really aggravate me, but now I keep reminding myself that he's scared, and this is the only way he knows how to show it. I try to remember that he's a really good kid when he's calm, and I take a breath before saying stuff to him, so I don't say something I'll regret."*
>
> —Educator (Blaustein & Kinniburgh, 2019)

Despite our best intentions, or proactive and preventive efforts, conflict and tension still occur in learning environments. Stressful and traumatic events cause emotional and behavioral escalation. In the face of any stressor, the body activates the stress response and circulates stress hormones that affect a variety of body functions. A severe stress response happens to everyone *sometimes*. Young people are more susceptible to poorly controlled escalation because they're still growing mechanisms to manage it. One effect of trauma is to "train" the body to activate the stress response more often and more intensely (Blaustein & Kinniburgh, 2019). Thus, helping students learn to de-escalate is helpful for all students and especially healing for students with trauma (Yule, Houston, & Grych, 2019).

Phases of escalation

Trauma-informed educators understand how students can be triggered into emotional and behavioral escalation, which changes their readiness to learn, as well as their coping approaches (Johnson, 2018; Thomas, 2017; Madea, 2018; Brunzell, Stokes, & Waters, 2016).

Calm and engaged: Many pedagogical engagement strategies assume that students are calm and engaged. In this phase, students are not escalated; rather, we tend to see them on task, following rules and meeting expectations and responsive to positive affirmation. They are usually excited to learn and initiate positive, socially constructive behavior. Within the brain, the cortex, or "active learning center," is responsive to engagement and challenges, including those that require planning, reasoning or logic, imagination and complex communication.

At this phase, students show focus, contentment, confidence, problem-solving and patience. They generally respond well to new information, big ideas and constructive feedback. Students who are calm and engaged easily make eye contact and are relaxed throughout their bodies. They also collaborate well and tend to have fun with large-scale projects, including in partners and groups.

Agitation: When triggered or stressed, students may first show agitation. As the body initiates the stress response, chemicals such as cortisol and adrenaline can interrupt the cortex. Agitated students find it challenging to access old memories and form new ones, establish and respect boundaries, understand consequences, inhibit their impulses or imagine constructive solutions. This phase is marked by students being distracted and switching between being off- and on-task as well as in and out of group or partner activities. Students may also leave their seat or space and talk with others about unrelated content or ideas.

Acceleration: If agitation is not resolved and a stressor is insufficiently addressed, students may accelerate. At this phase, stress hormones intensely call the brain away from active learning functions in the cortex and toward the midbrain, which is more responsible for things like emotions and visual and auditory processing. Students may show avoidance, withdrawal and escape behaviors, such as lack of eye contact, head on desk, covered ears, hunching or turning away. They may flush, with their skin turning red or darker. Their body may show tension, such as with veins emerging on the forehead or temple. Students exhibit high distractibility, such as asking tangential or unrelated questions. They often pair desirable behaviors with inappropriate ones and seek attention or confrontation, such as by arguing or using profanity. Overly simple thinking at this phase makes it difficult for students to perceive nuance and constructive options, so educators may hear language that suggests an "us vs. them" or "me vs. you" mentality.

Peak distress: At this phase, also called the "rage" phase, a student's stress hormones are disrupting the cortex, mid-brain and even brain stem. The brainstem is responsible for breathing, temperature regulation, hunger and thirst signals, raw alarm and threat assessment, as well as sleep routines. Students who reach peak distress may show extreme crying, clumsy and erratic movement, flushed skin, and ragged, rapid or irregular breathing, including hyperventilation. Enraged students minimally use and respond to language. They may shout, have rapid or incomplete speech and fail to answer clearly or at all to verbal prompts. Consistent with a severe stress response, students may try to run away or leave the situation. They may also make loud noises, aggressive suggestions or gestures, or attempt to destroy, which can include self-harm.

Recovery: As the body starts to process stress hormones, a student often takes a deep breath or a few gasping breaths. This signals the beginning of a return to equilibrium, not arrival to calm or readiness to learn. As students continue to de-escalate, their brains and bodies recover from the strain of the stress response. They may be fatigued, thirsty and strongly desire a chance to reconnect with a trusted adult. Cortisol can take up to five hours to return to baseline levels; water and a snack can help. In this phase, a student may be confused, wandering, staring, fidgeting or sleepy.

Contagious calm

For many educators, students' emotional and behavioral escalation is assumed to be misbehavior, a deliberate step away from the values and norms of the learning community. Such personal interpretations of behavior—that students are motivated to bother or deliberately upsetting daily goals, rather than reasonably responding to a perceived threat—usually triggers adult escalation (Souers & Hall, 2016; Venet, 2021). Reacting to these misconceptions often unfortunately further triggers students, creating a whirlwind of escalation, where each party mirrors and amplifies the other's distress.

Trauma-informed educators practice self-regulation, such as by incorporating mindful moments and grounding activities into their routines. Regular mindfulness practice helps increase the brief time between a stressor and an action, helping to transform educators from reactive to responsive (Jennings, 2015).

At every phase of escalation, trauma-informed educators invite students to mirror de-escalating, non-verbal strategies:

- Breathe deeply, deliberately and regularly.
- Connect with calm gaze that shows emotion.
- Disengage and decrease stimuli.
- Open and visible palms may indicate a willingness to listen and collaborate.
- Practice patience.
- Provide a warm, safe and comforting space.
- Relax jaw, eyes and shoulders.
- Stabilize your stance and take up appropriate space with your face, shoulders and hips pointing forward, and stay upright (this can include kneeling for easy eye contact).
- State boundaries simply.
- Vocalize authority with a low, resonant tone.

Reflections

- Imagine that one student has just demeaned another: What de-escalation tactics would you try?
- Think of a specific student who struggles with escalation. How might strategies like "relating" and "regulating" look in practice for them?

Recommended resource

"Understanding the Cycle of a Meltdown" by Cassandra Johnson, **oraeyc.org/single-post/2018/11/26/Understanding-the-Cycle-of-a-Meltdown**

Restorative practices

This section introduces practices to introduce and strengthen restorative justice in schools. Restorative and trauma-informed practices significantly overlap. They inform the entire course and especially the next few chapters, including "Stop bullying," "Discipline with dignity," "Interrupt shame," "Coordinate repentance" and "Encourage emotional literacy."

Schools have adopted a variety of restorative justice practices (Advancement Project, AFT, NEA, National Opportunity to Learn Campaign, 2014; Lodi, Perrella, Lepri, Scarpa, & Patrizi, 2022; Fronius, et al., 2019). Here, we briefly review restorative practices and interventions with attention to multi-tiered systems of support (Katic, Alba, & Johnson, 2020; Darling-Hammond S., 2023).

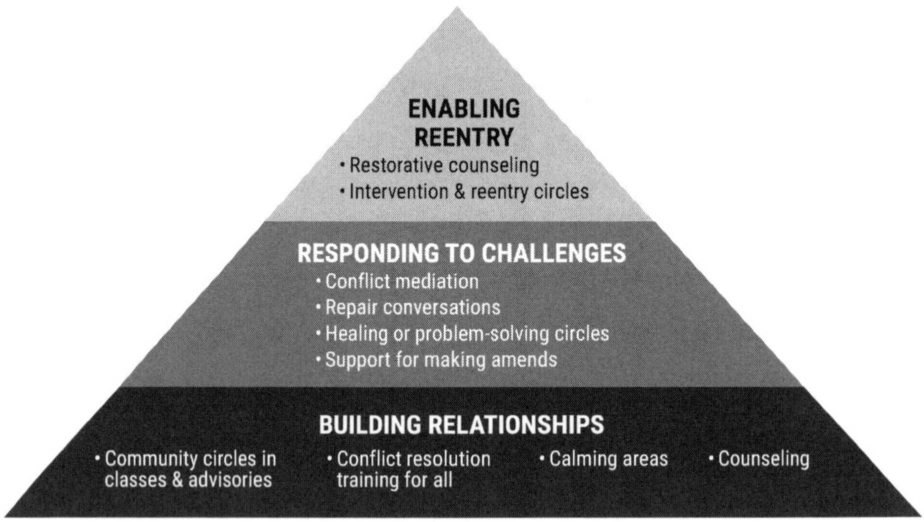

Restorative practices can be integrated into multi-tiered systems of support (Learning Policy Institute, 2023).

Tier 1 interventions focus on serving all students, all the time. They are often called "universal" and build core skills, as well as relationships. Some restorative practices that align with this tier include:

- **Adult mentorship**
- **Affective statements and questions** to reflect on feelings and how a particular behavior impacts others' feelings
- **Inclusive decision-making**

- **Preventive resolution programs** focus on building problem-solving and regulation skills. These programs teach students how to exercise self-control, diffuse a situation, assuage hurt feelings and reduce chances for retaliation after conflict
- **Social-emotional learning programs** focus on making safe, ethical choices and developing caring and positive relationships
- **Teaching apologies**

Tier 2 interventions tailor programming, such as to a smaller group within a school community, when Tier 1 strategies have not fully addressed a need. Tier 2 restorative practices include:

- **Peer mediation:** Trained student peers facilitate dialogue or restorative justice practices between students to address an issue and come to a solution to avoid future conflict. Collectively, mediation participants may discuss the norm or rule that was violated, who was affected, and how a referred student can repair it.
- **Role play** focuses on repentance or one of its components.

Tier 3 interventions are typically reserved for serious challenges and last resort measures if efforts at Tier 1 or Tier 2 were insufficient. They will likely require more time than interventions at Tier 1 or 2 and possibly more iterative revisiting of key concepts, skills, steps or expectations. For trauma-informed educators, Tier 3 restorative practices could look like:

- **Community service** allowing individuals to restore after harm committed to the school community by providing a meaningful service and contributing to their individual improvement or growth
- **Referral to a colleague or clinician** who may assess a student and/or offer more one-on-one, intensive support

Circle: A Flexible Restorative Practice

Circle process is a popular restorative approach that can be adapted for any tier. A circle is a facilitated meeting. Both seating in the round and explicit participation guidelines (which may require turn taking, active listening, explicit opt-in and opt-out from a discussion or topic and more) democratize contributions and aim to provide a safe environment for all. Educators use restorative circles for a wide range of aims, including:

- Celebrating successes
- Check-ins to open or end the day
- Delivering content instruction
- Developing relationships and building community
- Discussing concerns
- Problem solving
- Responding to wrong-doing and conflict
- Teaching listening and respect

Additionally, *restorative community conferences* may take place in a circle process. These facilitated meetings convene a wrongdoer and person(s) harmed, as well as other key stakeholders if needed, such as teachers and parents, to discuss the circumstances that led to harm and solutions.

Restorative justice programs, often by definition, change discipline outcomes in schools, such as reduced suspensions, expulsions and incident referrals (Fronius, et al., 2019; Katic, Alba, & Johnson, 2020). They are also linked to improvements in school climate, including belonging, emotional skills, equity and relationship quality; attendance rates; and academic outcomes (Lodi, Perrella, Lepri, Scarpa, & Patrizi, 2022).

Importantly, restorative practices reduce traumatic effects in those who were harmed, including by reducing avoidance coping and recurring, intrusive thoughts about the prior violation (Lloyd & Borrill, 2020). Furthermore, restorative practices are linked with improvements in children's health and well-being, including depression and anxiety (Lodi, Perrella, Lepri, Scarpa, & Patrizi, 2022). This may be because restorative practices boost protective factors such as social skills, self-esteem and positive social connections (Katic, Alba, & Johnson, 2020).

Finally, restorative practices represent a powerful tool for equitable outcomes among students, with the strongest positive effects seen among marginalized students (Darling-Hammond S., 2023). While restorative practices are most impactful in school communities that commit to systemic changes, every additional exposure to restorative practices is linked to improved student behavior, mental health and disciplinary outcomes (Darling-Hammond S., 2023).

17 Stop bullying

CONTENT NOTE. This chapter includes ideas related to bullying, homophobia and racism.

> *"Students want educators to recognize the signs of trauma and mental illness; they want schools to protect them from bullying and deal with it immediately if it occurs; and they want access to crisis counselors."*
>
> —Onyeka-Crawford, Patrick and Chaudhry (Let Her Learn: Stopping School Pushout for Girls of Color, 2017)

Schools are not consistently a "safe space" from violence and adversity, especially for marginalized students (Carlton, 2017; Petrone & Rogers Stanton, 2021). Bullying is the most common form of violence students face at school (Centers for Disease Control and Prevention, 2024). Trauma-informed educators recognize that schools can play a role in "causing and worsening trauma" (Venet, 2021). This chapter focuses on strategies to address violence at school and intervene in bullying.

Identify bullying

Educators are aware of more than 70 percent of the bullying incidents students experience, which generally takes one of four forms: (Wachs, Bilz, Niproschke, & Schubarth, 2018):

Verbal attacks, including hate speech, insults, name-calling, slurs, teasing and threats.

Physical behaviors, including beating, damaging targeted student's property, detaining, fighting, hitting, kicking and pushing.

Relational and social aggression, such as deliberate social exclusion and rumor-spreading.

Cyberbullying, such as using social media to amplify misinformation, or to develop an "outsider" narrative.

At least one in five students is bullied at school and 16 percent face cyberbullying (Centers for Disease Control and Prevention, 2024). Marginalized students are much more likely to be bullied and face violence at school (Irwin, Wang, Cui,

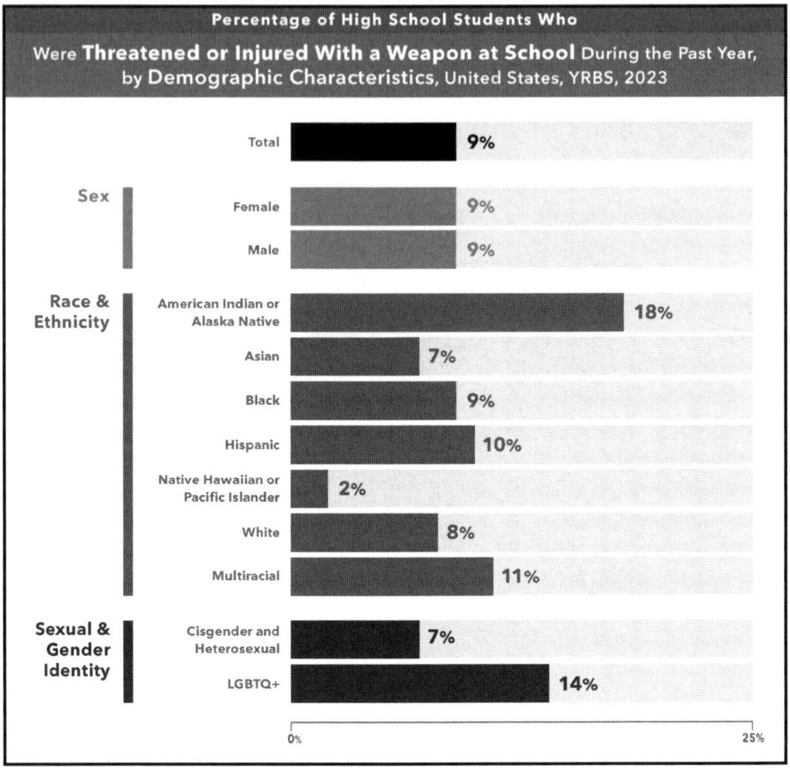

Percentages of high school students who were bullied at school during the past year, by demographic characteristics. Bar charts show that 19 percent of all students were bullied; 22 percent of female students were bullied compared to 17 percent of male students; 29 percent of LGBTQIA+ students were bullied compared to 16 percent of cisgender and heterosexual students (Centers for Disease Control and Prevention, 2024).

Zhang, & Thompson, 2021; Kurtz, Lloyd, Harwin, Comai, & Gong, 2024; Centers for Disease Control and Prevention, 2024). Some of the starkest disparities are between LGBTQIA+ students and their cisgender and heterosexual peers, with the former almost twice as likely to report being bullied as the latter.

- Some data suggest that bullying happens during instructional time: Most gay students say that their classmates' contributions in class "make it harder for me to learn" compared to just 1 in 3 of their heterosexual peers (Kurtz, Lloyd, Harwin, Comai, & Gong, 2024).
- Other data suggest that bullying contributes to chronic absenteeism among LGBTQIA+ students, who are twice as likely as cisgender peers to say they did not attend school in the past month because of safety concerns (Centers for Disease Control and Prevention, 2024).

Bullying is also associated with poor mental and physical health outcomes, lack of social relationships, economic hardships and decreased quality of life into adulthood (Fraguas, Diaz-Caneja, & Ayora, 2021; Lowry, Kennedy, & Johns, 2022).

Analyze power imbalances

Bullying may be best understood as "systematic abuse of power by peers" (Menesini & Salmivalli, 2017; Fraguas, Diaz-Caneja, & Ayora, 2021). A bully may derive power from physical strength, social status or group size, such as when a group targets a single person. Bullies may also leverage knowledge of a peer's vulnerabilities to wound. Targeted traits often center around difference from the group norm and/or taboos, and may be related to:

- Ethnic, racial, gender or sexual identity
- Family situation
- Learning challenges, learning disability and/or neurodivergence
- Migration or refugee status
- Personal characteristics or traits, such as appearance

Bullies tend to lack empathy and demonstrate a sense of self-importance and entitlement. They value dominance, are confident about using aggression and expect aggression to have positive outcomes, such as peer approval and educators' acceptance (Menesini & Salmivalli, 2017).

Effectively stop bullying

Up to 30 percent of students who have been the victim of bullying did not tell anyone due to shame. Support from adults is often essential and students expect educators to actively intervene when violence occurs at school—not observe, ignore, dismiss or trivialize it (Wachs, Bilz, Niproschke, & Schubarth, 2018). Unfortunately, educators inconsistently intervene to address bullying. They are more likely to address physical and verbal violence than relational or cyberbullying (Wachs, Bilz, Niproschke, & Schubarth, 2018). Educators are least likely to address bullying based on sexual orientation or gender identity (Irwin, Wang, Cui, Zhang, & Thompson, 2021; Wachs, Bilz, Niproschke, & Schubarth, 2018). Educators who intervene are effective in ending bullying—both in the short term and the long-term. Interventions can be grouped into three styles (Wachs, Bilz, Niproschke, & Schubarth, 2018).

Authoritarian strategies include efforts to expel, give students a "particular look," punish, suspend, threaten or withhold desired experience, such as a field trip or recess. These are common, yet minimally effective over time. Authoritarian approaches provide no positive model for social behaviors, create a negative class climate and increase covert and indirect bullying, which are more challenging to observe and stop. Educators who rely on hierarchy and deference to manage student behavior may unwittingly support the logic of dominance and aggression that informs bullying (Wachs, Bilz, Niproschke, & Schubarth, 2018).

Individual support strategies can look like talking to students who have bullied others, as well as talking to students who have been victimized to offer emotional support and gather information. These efforts are up to 1.6 times more likely to stop bullying than authoritarian approaches (Wachs, Bilz, Niproschke, & Schubarth, 2018). Yet "talking it out" may fail to consistently address peer power imbalances and generally do not build the skills of either the bully or the targeted student to behave differently when faced with a new opportunity.

> Cooperative support strategies are
> **up to 5X**
> more likely to stop bullying than punishment or authoritarian approaches
> (Wachs, Bilz, Niproschke, & Schubarth, 2018).

Cooperative support strategies include the whole group. "Whole group" is a flexible term and may reflect an entire class, all the students who ride the same bus, or even partnership with parents and other school staff. Cooperative support aims to change social dynamics and positively influence school climate. These approaches turn collective attention to resolving the challenge of inadequate connection, rather than the poor bond between any two or a few students and are up to five times more likely to stop bullying than punishment or authoritarian approaches (Wachs, Bilz, Niproschke, & Schubarth, 2018). To effectively address bullying, trauma-informed educators (Wachs, Bilz, Niproschke, & Schubarth, 2018; Fraguas, Diaz-Caneja, & Ayora, 2021; Menesini & Salmivalli, 2017; Kaba, 2021):

- Actively practice empathy and support for marginalized people and targeted students.
- Clearly communicate disapproval of bullying behaviors.
- Explain the concept of a "bystander."
- Prepare students as peer educators and assertive supporters.
- Reward collaboration over dominance or aggression.
- Support friendships and positive peer relationships, especially for marginalized students.

Reflections

- How might you increase students' willingness to ask for help with bullying?
- Which bullying intervention style best aligns with what you typically do?

Recommended resource

"Bullying Intervention in Schools: A Multilevel Analysis of Teachers' Success in Handling Bullying from the Students' Perspective" by Sebastian Wachs, Ludwig Bilz, Sasia Niproschke and Wilfried Schubarth, **sci-hubst/10.1177/0272431618780423**

18 Discipline with dignity

CONTENT NOTE. This chapter includes ideas related to mental illness, policing, racism and shame.

> *"Violence is an option if you're powerful and can hit hard and get away with it."*
>
> —Ellen Reddy (Mathewson, 2022)

Restorative practices reflect a whole-school relational approach to building school climate and addressing student behavior that fosters belonging over exclusion, social engagement over control, and meaningful accountability over punishment. This chapter expands on the previous one, "Stop bullying" and challenges trauma-informed educators to critically reflect on the impacts of authoritarian discipline, as well as opportunities for more effective and ethical ways to facilitate learning environments.

Live by principles

Trauma-informed initiatives often lead with facts, figures and science. Conversely, restorative justice is rooted in global Indigenous wisdom, traditions and principles such as "Violations create new obligations, through which justice and relational balance can be restored" and "All parties involved in a conflict have needs to consider" (Lodi, Perrella, Lepri, Scarpa, & Patrizi, 2022). Furthermore, restorative practices are historically grounded in values (Evans & Vaandering, 2016; High, 2017), such as:

- Belonging
- Collaboration
- Encouragement
- Equality
- Honesty
- Interconnectedness
- Personal worth and well-being
- Support
- Trust
- Wholeness and healing

Approaching students' undesirable behaviors with attention to values provides a flexible foundation for trauma-informed educators to exercise creativity and compassion in thinking about conflict prevention and resolution.

Critically reflect: Punishment and policing tactics

"Punishment excludes and excises.
It demolishes relationships and community."
—Stephanie Foo (What My Bones Know: A Memoir of Healing from Complex Trauma, 2022)

Though few educators still espouse a belief in "zero tolerance," exclusionary punishment that is excessive, inequitable, minimally justified or justifiable and that undermines educational progress is increasingly popular (Curren, 2020). One possible root cause is the widespread idea that people must feel bad (e.g., experience shame or suffering or cruelty) in order to change or improve undesirable behavior (Walker, Tarutani, & Furman, 2017; Kaba, 2021). Punishment-based disciplinary models assume that children's undesirable behaviors are best treated as intentional insubordination, criminal infractions, subversion or delinquency, rather than efforts at coping or communicating (Curren, 2020). They also insist that adults regulate and direct student behavior—and therefore lack "effective processes [for students] to learn and repair harm" (Walker, Tarutani, & Furman, 2017). These models interrupt classroom relationship building by isolating compliant, calm and obedient students from those whose struggles are more defiant or outwardly challenging. Rather than helping to establish accountability or guiding behavior change, these tactics deepen social fractures by drawing boundaries around who it's okay to harm and when.

Longstanding disciplinary models are based on law enforcement, such as by requiring the same reaction to every problem, no matter the circumstance(s) or root cause(s) (National Women's Law Center, 2016; Curren, 2020). But policing behaviors—including coercion, control, incapacitation, isolation, punishment and surveillance—are not limited to law enforcement officers; we find these tactics in many fields that touch children's lives (Roberts, 2022).

Impacts of policing tactics

Wherever we find them, policing tactics are ineffective. Like other traumatic events, policing undermines trust and leads to hypervigilance (Smith Lee & Robinson, 2019), as well as significant stress, feelings of powerlessness, disrespect, shame, fear and judgment (Schmidt, Stretten, & Briscoe, 2021). Repeated exposure to school policing is a "potent predictor" of heightened emotional distress and post-traumatic stress symptoms, with students of color consistently reporting that policing makes them feel less safe (Jackson, Fahmy, Vaughn, & Testa, 2019; Rollins & Thomas, 2020). Policing tactics do not just lead to unpleasant feelings. Like other forms of violence and childhood adversity, increased exposure to police is also linked to traumatic effects, including adverse mental health (Schmidt, Stretten, & Briscoe, 2021; Bor, Venkataramani, Williams, & Tsai, 2018) and reduced academic performance, with policing negating the benefits of core educational interventions (Legewie & Fagan, 2019).

Discrimination and disparity

Traditional discipline models are harmful for all students. They are also discriminatory—levying harms disproportionately against some students more than others. From preschool through high school, children of color and especially Black students receive "more complaints about their behavior and recommendations for disciplinary action" (Sabol, et al., 2022). Importantly, researchers attribute these disparate outcomes to educator bias and not actual differences in the rates of students' undesirable behaviors. Increased rates of preschool educators' complaints about student behavior are associated with lower grades, absenteeism and disengagement with school in later years (Sabol, et al., 2022). In fact, experiencing traumatic events—including exposure to domestic violence, living with a parent struggling with mental illness, exposure to adult substance abuse, being physically victimized, having an incarcerated parent or just being in a severely poor household—increases students' odds of being suspended or expelled by 80 percent (Zeng, Corr, O'Grady, & Guan, 2019). Researchers have also found that children who have been hit, children who are involved with child protective services and those participating in programs for free and reduced-price school meals are all more likely to be suspended than their peers (Sanders, et al., 2024). In contrast, schools and educators that use trauma-informed and restorative practices narrow disparities in discipline outcomes by race and disability status; reduce isolation tactics like suspension and expulsion; improve student attendance and academic performance; improve school climate; and reduce educators' compassion fatigue while improving their retention and satisfaction (Educator Policy and Innovation Center, 2017; Fronius, et al., 2019).

Experiencing traumatic events increases students' odds of being suspended or expelled by

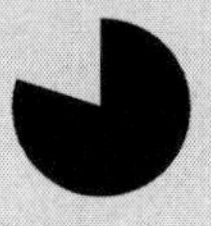

80%

(Zeng, Corr, O'Grady, & Guan, 2019).

Leverage consequences

Trauma-informed educators pursue students' well-being and an ethical school community. They focus on treating behavior challenges as important learning opportunities rather than key moments to flex authority. This requires elevating relationships and dialogue, creative problem-solving, restorative practices and community service (Curren, 2020). When appropriate, leverage two types of consequences:

- Natural consequences occur without adult intervention. Trauma-informed educators observe natural consequences and take opportunities to motivate reflection and new skill development. For example, if a student is playing during a meal and spills part of it onto a now-sticky floor, you might ask, "How did that happen? Can you help me make sure this doesn't make anybody trip or fall? What might you do differently next time?"

- Logical consequences rely on reasonable, related and respectful intervention that reinforces a student's existing skills. For example, if a student is making taunting remarks to a peer, you might interrupt by saying something like, "This sounds like bullying and that's not okay. I'm counting on you to share kindness and care. Let's take turns celebrating instead of put downs—I'll go first. I love that you __. Your turn: I would like to hear you celebrate or say something kind about [the student they targeted]."

Consequences may be uncomfortable or even unpleasant. They should also clearly relate to the problem at hand and focus on existing strengths and expectations, rather than cruelty or pain.

Reflection

- In the 1990s, the developmental needs of misbehaving youth were dismissed with the phrase "adult time for adult crime" (Curren, 2020). Develop a pithy phrase in support of trauma-informed practices and/or restorative justice.
- Review High's reflections on sharing circles in a K–8 Illinois district (2017). How might the "essential elements of dignity" inform Tier 2 or Tier 3 restorative justice programming in your school community?

Recommended resource

"Using Restorative Practices to Teach and Uphold Dignity in an American School District" by Anna High, **id.erudit.org/iderudit/1044479ar**

19 Interrupt shame

CONTENT NOTE. This chapter includes ideas related to shame.

> *"Trauma leads to shame. Trauma determines the content of shame. Shame pushes the body into a traumatic response. The more I learn about the two, the more I am convinced of their deep connection to one another."*
>
> —Lucia Osborne-Crowley (How shame makes us sick, 2020)

Exploring emotions and practicing effective coping can help to prevent an adverse or traumatic event from becoming a traumatic experience by ending or mitigating the stress response. Trauma-informed educators also understand shame as a critical emotional experience that is "inextricably linked" with developing traumatic effects (Thiesen-Womersley, 2021).

Complicate "synonyms"

Some human emotions are only experienced in social settings—or when we perceive that we are "seen"—including guilt, humiliation, pride and shame. Some of these emotional labels are used interchangeably. Relatedly, many people assume that both guilt and shame are useful to inhibit illegal, immoral or interpersonally harmful behavior ... but guilt and shame are *not* equally useful for social settings and behavior change. Shame and guilt have very different effects on behavior, well-being and lasting traumatic effects (Tangney, 2008).

Guilt is the sense that one's actions are wrong, that one has made a mistake. Conversely, "We feel shame when [...] when some part of our core self is perceived to be inadequate, inappropriate, or immoral" (Dolezal & Gibson, 2022). Shame is an intense, internalized emotional experience that fundamentally threatens and overwhelms a healthy sense of self. It can also tip the scale from a young person perceiving a traumatic event as 'a bad thing happened to me' to 'proof that I'm a bad person' (Tangney, 2008).

Shame hurts

Shame can provoke powerful feelings of despair, inferiority, powerlessness, defectiveness and self-contempt (Dolezal & Gibson, 2022). In the moment, shame is often unbearable. Shame begets more shame, so most people go to great lengths to avoid it, including by acting out and projecting their poor self-image onto others as anger and aggression (Tangney, 2008). Avoidance and defensive behaviors can also include apathy, depression, perfectionism, narcissism and withdrawal (Dolezal & Gibson, 2022). In fact, shame defenses are nearly identical to common acute trauma responses:

- **Flight:** flee, avoid, change the subject
- **Fight:** double down, make accusations, get aggressive
- **Freeze:** deny involvement, crumble when confronted

Shame amplifies negative emotions and is an important indicator that a stressful or traumatic event will have lasting, traumatic effects (López-Castro, Saraiya, Zumberg-Smith, & Dambreville, 2019). In fact, while both guilt and shame are associated with post-traumatic stress symptoms, shame is the more powerful predictor (Shi, Ren, Zhao, & Chan, 2021).

Spot shame

Directly confronting a student who is actively experiencing shame may escalate, rather than resolve, a school conflict. However, trauma-informed educators are sensitive to shame because it can distort learning, thwart healing and transform one student's lack of psychological safety into a physical safety issue for others. People who experience shame may show several different types of signs, including (Livingstone, 2020; Dolezal & Gibson, 2022):

- Trying to withdraw, hide or disappear: averted eye contact, blushing or flushing, covered face, pulling away
- Negative self-talk or descriptions with terms like "self-conscious, embarrassed, foolish, worthless, inept or inferior"
- Speech markers that signal avoidance like stammering, silence, or long pauses

Shame at school

Shame has a long history in schools. First, because adults have so much power over students as subordinates (Salter & Hall, 2020). Second, because shame requires an audience, which is easy to find in schools (Stearns & Stearns, 2016). And finally, because shame was once seen as an improved classroom management strategy over corporal punishment (Stearns & Stearns, 2016). Besides jeopardizing learning, shame-based practices threaten to legitimize and entrench inequity (Salter & Hall, 2020). Trauma-informed educators critically reflect on their own practice and school cultures to identify behaviors and circumstances that are likely to lead to shame, such as:

- Belittling labels for failure to perform normatively
- Open criticism; statements and observations made to rebuke

- Required physical differentiation from peers—such as by changing locations, clothing or posture—thereby encouraging ridicule
- Required vulnerability—such as about bodies, families, health or lifestyle—that does not enthusiastically uphold students' inherent value
- Stigmatizing language and/or holding students accountable for circumstances that may be more structural than personal or that reflect an effort to cope with adversity
- Withholding opportunities, such as to participate in recess or attend a field trip (Stearns & Stearns, 2016; Salter & Hall, 2020; Dolezal & Gibson, 2022)

Validation, choice and support help students regulate shame-based responses. Positive interactions can help tamp down shame in learning environments. Focusing on effort and perseverance instead of perfection or mastery can help students shift from mindsets rooted in fear to ones that affirm and value growth processes.

Affirm dignity

Early shame researchers advocated transforming shame into the more effective guilt. Guilt, again, motivates remorse and behavior change, includes more emotional space for recognizing mistakes without internalizing them as inherent flaws, and undergirds more impactful accountability efforts: "Guilt is the 'better way to feel bad'" (Tangney, 2008).

With a deep appreciation for how trauma and shame are "inextricably linked" (Thiesen-Womersley, 2021), some advocate not just for strategies to manage and mitigate shame, but to deliberately foster its opposite: dignity. To achieve and affirm dignity, trauma-informed educators acknowledge both the inherent value of young people and human vulnerability to shame and injury (Salter & Hall, 2020; Dolezal & Gibson, 2022). This work includes:

- Emotional and physical regulation
- Empathy and relation, including without judgment, criticism or ridicule, to accept and understand the presence of the feeling of shame
- Reasoning about the harmful behavior, self-kindness and natural consequences
- Directly combatting sociopolitical causes of shame and trauma

Reflections

- Can you think of a time as a child when you broke a rule or failed to meet an expectation and a caring adult emotionally connected, clearly explained why your behavior was unacceptable or dangerous and helped you prepare to change for next time? How did that feel? Did you repair the wrong?

- Can you think of an example of the opposite: When you were shamed? Do you remember learning anything constructive from that experience?

Recommended resource

"Beyond a trauma-informed approach and towards a shame-sensitive practice" by Luna Dolezal and Matthew Gibson, **nature.com/articles/s41599-022-01227-z.pdf**

20 Coordinate repentance

CONTENT NOTE. This chapter includes ideas related to shame.

> *"[Repentance is] a kind of self-care. [...] We give attention to our own broken places, our own reactionary impulses, our own careless ignorance. 'Facing the harm I caused is an act of profound optimism. It is a choice to grow, to learn, to become someone who is more open and empathetic.' Making amends also calls on us to put real things at stake, to take real risks, and to 'pull up anchors that might make it all too easy to repeat past behaviors.'"*
>
> —Rabbi Danya Ruttenberg (2022)

In this section, we've examined the science of restoration—including facilitating cooperative support, affirming dignity and preventing shame. Another critical component of restorative practice is repair after conflict, harm and tension. In this chapter, we focus on repentance—especially good apologies—as a key restorative practice.

Judaism is one example of a cultural and faith tradition that advocates a restorative approach to prepare children to live in thoughtful community, especially after harm. Rabbi Danya Ruttenberg (2022) writes of three components of the concept of restoration, with attention to different stakeholders:

- **Atonement:** reconciliation, an action (option) left 'up to God'
- **Forgiveness:** a conscious, deliberate choice of the person(s) harmed to release resentment and/or vengeance
- **Repentance:** a process by the person(s) who committed harm

Repentance is a process

Punishment depends on an authority figure deciding what will resolve a situation and enforcing compliance, often quickly. A restorative approach is more demanding. It requires more stakeholders to reflect, grow and act, often by consensus. Repentance may take longer and often demands an orchestra of skills: emotional and behavioral regulation, emotional literacy, effective communication, empathy and perspective-taking, problem-solving, compromise and solidarity.

Trauma-informed educators iteratively help students with each of those component skills, as well as the specific skills to achieve repentance (Kaba & Hayes, 2021; Clarren, 2023; Ruttenberg, 2022):

1. Stop doing the harm.
2. Acknowledge: Name and own the full harm perpetrated and accept consequences.
3. Start to change: Become the kind of person who doesn't do harm, which requires significant inner work.
4. Restore: Make amends for harm done, in whatever way possible.
5. Repair: Apologize for the harm caused to make your relationship as right as possible with the person(s) harmed.
6. When presented with the opportunity, make different choices and new mistakes.

Evaluate apologies

Apologies are often a demand of a punishment model. Without a full repentance process, apologies can entrench power imbalances: One party has the power to decide when and whether to apologize; the other party must wait for it. Power imbalances also mean that apologies can be misused (Thobani, 2023; Zoodsma & Schaafsma, 2022):

- Apologies can manipulate and coerce assimilation. For example, apologies that a person offers because they want to be more accepted, rather than to transform or address the circumstances that informed a violation.
- Apologies can be self-serving, making the apologizer feel better, even if a full repentance process is not complete or underway.
- Apologies can produce a backlash, such as by challenging social or shared conceptions of who or what caused harm, and who must be accountable.
- Apologies can fail to fundamentally transform relationships in favor of solidifying the status quo. For instance, by choosing what to include in an apology, it is possible to obscure and avoid accountability for select elements of a violation.

By themselves, words and gestures may not be sufficient to constitute an effective apology. Still, as outlined above, apology is a critical step in the repentance process. Importantly, the other components of repentance should be done *with* the harmed (at least in spirit) and not *to* them (Ruttenberg, 2022). Done well, apologies can promote healing, address shame and restore relationships (Walker, Tarutani, & Furman, 2017).

Reflections

- "The power of the word sorry from an adult to a student is palpable. It's an act often met by surprised student faces because the humanity behind an adult or authority figure admitting fault is hard to miss" (Pickens, 2020). How can you introduce, encourage and model effective apologies among students?
- How can you regularly foster a culture of relationship and habits of repair?

Recommended resource

"Repentance, Repair, and What True Forgiveness Takes: Lessons from Maimonides for the Modern World" by Maria Popova, **themarginalian.org/2022/10/24/repentance-repair-ruttenberg**

21 Encourage emotional literacy

CONTENT NOTE. This chapter includes ideas related to racism and suicide.

> *"Being healed is about feeling the appropriate emotions at the appropriate times and still being able to come back to yourself."*
>
> —Stephanie Foo (What My Bones Know: A Memoir of Healing from Complex Trauma, 2022)

Every part of the restorative justice model demands emotional regulation and prosocial engagement. Furthermore, Ginwright (2018) holds emotional literacy and SEL central to healing-centered engagement. The Collaborative for Academic, Social, and Emotional Learning (CASEL) established an influential framework to break related growth into component skills and guide educators as they in turn support students. CASEL outlined five competencies: self-awareness, self-management, social awareness, relationship skills and responsible decision-making. Students in SEL programs strengthen targeted skills and competencies, improve relationships and social behaviors, reduce emotional distress and unwanted behaviors, and increase academic engagement and performance (Greenberg, 2023). Others find that SEL competencies directly address youth mental health and reduce the risk of suicide (Posamentier, Seibel, & DyTang, 2022).

Get curious

After a stressful or traumatic event, a young person might feel any emotion—or combination of them—including angry, fearful, hopeless, hysterical, irritable, jumpy, out of control, sad, uncertain, wary, worried ... A trauma-informed educator encourages emotional agency and helps students practice curiosity about their emotions with questions such as:

- What do you feel?
- How do those emotions influence or inform you?
- What can you do to change or manage these emotions?

Emotions can be complex

Accurately identifying emotions helps students learn and practice effective regulation strategies (López-Pérez & Pacella, 2021). Trauma-informed educators assist students with naming feelings by developing emotional vocabulary. Address both increasing complexity, such as blended emotions, and intensity, such as during times of great stress and transition. Words and verbal exchanges are just one way to show or assess emotional literacy and vocabulary. Nonverbal students, such as those with autism, benefit from emotional interventions that leverage dance, movement, art, music, drama and play. Such somatic, or body-oriented, interventions are often at the root of deep, satisfying social connections (Vulcan, 2021).

Emotions influence and inform

Beyond labeling, trauma-informed educators help students learn about and manage emotions and interactions. Emotional management includes using emotions as information. Consider some examples:

- **Fear** tells us to be cautious and vigilantly assess risk. It also invites us to be strategic, plan to overcome and work with others to solve problems. Fear might also push us to withdraw or lash out.
- **Joy** encourages us to live mindfully, without attention to past or future, but in the moment. It helps form lasting memories and reveals the kinds of things we might want to pursue to continue to have a satisfactory life. Joy can also escalate to overexcitement, which makes it harder to realistically assess what's happening around us and respond intentionally.
- **Disgust** influences us to avoid and finish things quickly. It encourages us to learn to live with unpleasant sensations and control our physical reactions. Disgust could also lead to hurtful choices, such as if we confuse a disgusting thing with a disgusting person or group.
- **Anger** can reveal our expectations and boundaries—usually because they have been disregarded or violated. It can spur us to clear communication and to evaluate how we exist in responsible relationships with others. Anger might also push us toward aggression and competition, which can instead increase our social distance from others and move us away from conflict resolution.

Change and regulate emotions

Once students identify how an emotion influences their default reactions and behaviors, they can select coping strategies that align with their goals. For example, students may choose to be present with their emotion, observing how it changes in intensity over time. Mindfulness techniques may help make this practice non-judgmental and productive.

Students may also choose to change their feelings, such as by visualizing a remote control and 'switching channels' in their brain to reframe something challenging or negative into something that proves their resilience and fortitude. Relaxation strategies, like controlled breathing and deliberate movement of the body's largest muscles, can also help students transform their feeling (Simmons-Duffin, 2018).

Finally, students might decide to explore the feeling in a new way, such as by using outrage about an injustice to talk with others and create a plan for change.

Inequitable expectations, unjust outcomes

Consider these statements: *We accommodate masculine anger and regulate masculine sadness. We eagerly seek out children's joy and talk them out of disappointment. Black neutrality is misread as anger; Black jubilation is misread as aggression.*

These statements may seem oversimplified, but emotional detection, expression and regulation are all related to systemic oppression. For example, teachers-in-training are more likely to falsely read Black children's faces as angry than their white counterparts (Halberstadt, et al., 2020). Such distorted perceptions of which emotions are present or appropriate for a given student to express contribute to disciplinary disparities and dislocation from school (Blake & Epstein, 2019). Furthermore, repression makes emotional regulation and processing nearly impossible, pushing people who cannot feel, or who are not allowed to feel, toward maladaptive coping and related health challenges (Valdez, 2023).

Full emotional expression is a form of freedom that is not always available to students at school. Trauma-informed educators critically reflect on the ways that systemic oppression contributes to conceptions of and expectations for emotional literacy. Two important realizations should inform work with students on emotional literacy: First, like other skills, emotional literacy develops over time; explicit instruction and support are essential to growth when students struggle with expectations for emotional expression or regulation (Sanchis-Sanchis, Grau, Moliner, & Morales-Murillo, 2020; López-Pérez & Pacella, 2021).

Second, some emotional regulation strategies mitigate systemic oppression. For example, Black parents often aim to reduce their children's public expressions of anger and fear, because these emotions are punished. Without context on how this is a circumstantial, or "sometimes" strategy to mitigate racism, Black children experience signs of toxic stress. Conversely, being honest with Black children—even as young as five and six years old—that such emotional repression is one way to cope with and navigate an unfair world can help them calmly practice target approaches. Importantly, trauma-informed educators examine opportunities to change the root causes of racialized emotional repression and other disparities, rather than counting on students to buffer or protect against their own oppression (Dunbar, Zeytinoglu, & Leerkes, 2023).

Reflections

How often do you deliberately integrate opportunities to practice social or emotional competencies into your work with students?

Recommended resource

"Trauma, Anger, Grief, & Healing: A Portrait of an Elementary Classroom" by Carolina Valdez, **https://journals.library.appstate.edu/index.php/JTSE/article/view/287?articlesBySimilarityPage=1**

Collective healing

Whole-school and whole-district approaches look beyond the skills of a single educator and toward coordinated, collective action to both prevent trauma and promote healing. This section introduces key tenets of trauma-informed institutional change that inform the entire course and especially the next few chapters, including "Embrace the whole school, whole community, whole child," "Champion the common good," "Effectively engage families" and "Institutionalize mandated support."

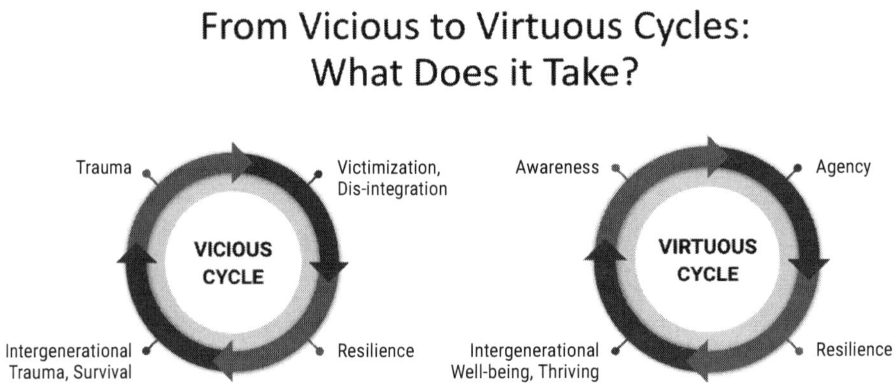

Virtuous cycles of intergenerational well-being depend on awareness and agency for thriving (Bass, et al., 2023).

Nurture virtuous cycles

Trauma-informed institutions acknowledge the ways that institutions—not just individuals within them—can harm and proactively endeavor to establish new dynamics. Like individual trauma, institutional trauma often leads to dysfunctional or maladaptive coping. Trauma flows through relational connections to be amplified and too often, trapped. Traumatizing institutions may:

- Dismiss past injustices as irrelevant.
- Misuse or withhold information to stigmatize.
- Reinforce or celebrate numbness in the face of heart-wrenching circumstances.
- Shame a group of people as inherently irrelevant, defective, inferior or "broken."

- Fragment funding flows, protocols and policy responses into smaller and smaller parts until it's almost impossible to see and serve the bigger picture.
- Show a persistent pattern of mistrust, territoriality or lack of cooperation (Calderon de la Barca, Milligan, & Kania, 2024).

In contrast, a trauma-informed institution aims to establish a virtuous cycle. That includes an appreciation for the 'fractal' nature of trauma and how it impacts individuals and collectives; ethically managed agency for all stakeholders; resilience, processing and healing practices; and ultimately, thriving (Bass, et al., 2023).

Powerfully collaborate

Whether stakeholders aim to improve a single student's academic outcomes, strengthen the role of caregivers or change an institution, relational connections are instrumental to success. Collaboration can be complicated because it implies shared power and active participation from diverse stakeholders in conceptualizing, planning and executing projects or shifts (Woo, LeTendre, Byun, & Schussler, 2022). Yet well-being and healing begin with small groups of committed, intentional actors whose efforts radiate effects outward to larger coalitions (Calderon de la Barca, Milligan, & Kania, 2024; Bass, et al., 2023).

Center the marginalized

"Many of our problems are social, structural and practical problems that stem from the idea that disabled people are fundamentally flawed, unworthy of inclusion, broken or inadequate. This is ableist thinking!"
–Ashley Shew (Against Technoableism: Rethinking Who Needs Improvement, 2023)

Systems redesign requires slow and deliberate strategies (Shapiro, 2021; Carter, Blanch, & Andrea, 2019). Shifting can be hard because "The more traumatized a system is, the more it will resist healing" (Calderon de la Barca, Milligan, & Kania, 2024). Directly addressing power imbalances is one of the most challenging things for school systems to undertake as they move toward trauma-informed models (Carter, Blanch, & Andrea, 2019). Trauma-informed educators practice centering these processes around the most vulnerable to shift who is marginalized and how. Return to questions such as:

- How do we know who is marginalized or most vulnerable?
- Are we challenging or extending the levers by which people in our collective become, and stay, marginalized or most vulnerable?
- How well are we promoting physical and psychological safety with the marginalized and most vulnerable?
- How can we (re)center around the needs of the marginalized and most vulnerable?

Acknowledging systemic trauma and achieving collective healing depends on our ability to recognize the silence and shaming that often come with power and dominant positions, as well as to undertake the hard work of undoing and redesigning. This is true of interpersonal bonds—and true of schools as institutions.

22 Campaign for the whole child

CONTENT NOTE. This chapter is not likely to upset or trigger readers with references to specific forms of harm.

> *"Those strategies are not just for school. Those strategies are for life."*
>
> —Andrea Mercer, assistant principal (Whole Child Model, 2024)

Schools in the 21st century do much more than facilitate academic growth; they are also children's health institutions. The conditions for effective learning are not just the responsibility of teachers or paraprofessionals. Rather, for students to be challenged, engaged, healthy, safe and supported at school, adults with diverse skill sets must coordinate policy, processes and practices. This chapter reviews whole-school approaches.

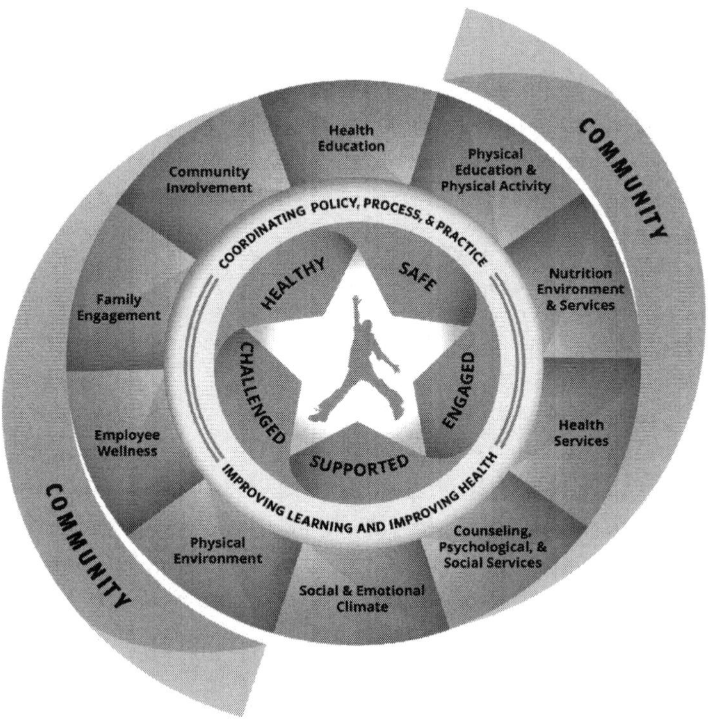

The Whole School, Whole Community, Whole Child model outlines a collaborative approach to learning and health with 10 total domains.

WSCC model

In 1987, a seminal article introduced the coordinated school health (CSH) model, a systems approach with eight domains for health promotion. CSH resonated with public health professionals working with and in schools, but less so with the education sector. Later, ASCD introduced the whole child model with five tenets to guide policy and programming. In 2013, ASCD and the U.S. Centers for Disease Control and Prevention partnered to align these models, establishing the Whole School, Whole Community, Whole Child (WSCC, pronounced like "whisk") model (Lewallen, Hunt, Potts-Datema, Zaza, & Giles, 2015).

Community schools

The community schools strategy structures processes and partnerships to achieve the WSCC model. This site-based strategy focuses on schools as a hub where students and families access resources they need to be successful in school and life. Community schools utilize partnerships to coordinate access to on-site, wraparound services aligned with student and family needs. Buildings are often open before school, after school, on weekends and through summers. Common aspects of community schools are integrated student supports, expanded learning time and opportunities, family and community engagement, and collaborative leadership and practice. To pull it all together, community schools rely on full-time staff coordinators who organize, strengthen bonds, convene stakeholders for democratic leadership and decision-making, oversee needs assessment and iterative evaluation, and plan for sustainability and continuous improvement (Bloodworth & Horner, 2019). Furthermore, community schools commit to organizational and cultural shifts to democratize the school with iterative input from diverse stakeholders (Stefanski, Valli, & Jacobson, 2016).

Community schools reduce disparities and improve student and community outcomes such as increased attendance, academic achievement and graduation rates (Maier, Daniel, Oakes, & Lam, 2017). The model is also cost-effective; one study estimated that a community schools coordinator can leverage each dollar invested to deliver an average of over seven dollars in valuable services and supports to families (Bloodworth & Horner, 2019).

Trauma-informed schools

Trauma-informed schools are interested in how WSCC components intersect with psychological well-being. There is no set of "rules" or single "definition" for a trauma-informed school (Maynard, Farina, Dell, & Kelly, 2019). Still, whether implementing Support for Students Exposed to Trauma, Cognitive Behavioral Intervention for Trauma in Schools, The Missouri Model or another framework, trauma-informed approaches operate with common principles and goals (Guarino & Chagnon, 2018; Baker, et al., 2020; Cook & Black, 2020; Parameswaran, Molloy, & Kuttner, 2023):

- Believe that healing happens in relationships.
- Ensure emotional, behavioral, academic, social and physical safety for all.
- Practice cultural and linguistic competence.
- Prevent retraumatization.
- Regularly use practices that promote trustworthiness, peer support, belonging, collaboration and critical reflection.
- Support agency, autonomy, choice, control and empowerment for students, staff and families.
- Understand trauma and its impact on brains, bodies and behaviors.
- View students holistically.

Training is essential to trauma-informed schools because trained educators improve their knowledge and confidence in novel practices (Sonsteng-Person & Loomis, 2021). Trauma-informed schools also improve student outcomes by reducing symptoms of post-traumatic stress and depression and by increasing desirable student behaviors and boosting student achievement (Berger, 2019).

Step-by-step to success

Schools can achieve robust implementation of novel whole-school models within three to five years (Cook & Black, 2020; Carter, Blanch, & Andrea, 2019; Partnership for the Future of Learning). Several tools guide exploration, planning, implementation and evaluation (The Center for Health and Healthcare in Schools, 2018; AFT, 2020). Here, we cover common steps and key questions.

Groundwork: Whether the goal is to improve student health outcomes, uptake of trauma-informed practices or connections to families, diverse stakeholders need to develop a shared understanding early.

- **Develop awareness:** All stakeholders need shared definitions and understanding to embed key ideas into informal conversation.

  Consider addressing questions such as: Can all school staff easily explain how trauma affects brains, bodies and behaviors? Do families share a general appreciation for the scientific basis that guides this work?

- **Evaluate urgency:** Foundational research can help to clarify challenges that are substantive enough to require institutional change.

  Consider addressing questions such as: Why is this important? Why should people commit to change now?

Plan to sustain: Provide a solid foundation. Institutions also typically reflect a complex tangle of laws, protocols, habits and beliefs. Investigating and even critically reflecting on policy, financial and ideological logistics must influence and inform opportunities and next steps.

- **Acknowledge barriers:** Misconceptions, tight budgets, limits on the allowable uses of funding and turnover are just some of the reasons that shared values and shared goals fail to come to fruition. Visually map the positions, relationships and patterns of influence in the school community to identify who holds significant influence.

  Consider addressing questions such as: What challenges your school community in moving forward? What gaps can be quickly addressed? What needs long-term attention and planning? Which people or organizations have something to gain (or lose) if your campaign is successful?

- **Assess readiness and resources:** Find champions, experts and co-conspirators who are prepared to lead. Analyze budgets, spaces, data, partners in other sectors, grant opportunities and skill sets to identify existing strengths and assets that can support staff, students and families through a change process. Investigate peer-reviewed research, high-quality books, clearinghouses and case studies that may help to inform which interventions are selected.

  Consider addressing questions such as: What do we hope to achieve? What do we know and do already? Who else needs to contribute to the vision of how this might be successful?

Mobilize and innovate: Try evidence-based, culturally relevant interventions. Seek feedback to tweak and adapt as new needs and issues arise.

- **Schedule a cycle:** Anticipate starting small. Plan to form and/or strengthen relationships for solidarity and progress. Set times and spaces to check in and follow up with diverse stakeholders.

  Consider addressing questions such as: How will the people we intend to support provide feedback and guide decisions about how well this serves their needs?

- **Iteratively intensify for impact:** Testing trauma-informed strategies is one of the most powerful ways educators can shift and sustain professional practice. Book study, small group reflections, peer observation, training and surveys are some of the ways to diversify school staff's continued engagement with concepts and skills. Calendar key opportunities for dialogue, reflection, evaluation and environmental review.

  Consider addressing questions such as: Whose comfort, convenience and experiences are centered in the current design? What new wrinkles have arisen in implementation? How can we measure our efforts? How will we know when and whether we have accomplished shared goals?

Celebrate and sustain: Ideally, the school community deepens awareness, sensitivity, responsiveness and justice-oriented practice to prevent and address trauma. These efforts should engage widening networks of community, stakeholders and audiences, such as to tell the story of growth, to advise others and to benefit from novel perspectives on institutional work.

- **Communicate success:** Message successes and lessons learned to establish and sustain trust, transparency and accountability. Share narratives to generate support and emphasize positive outcomes.

  Consider addressing questions such as: Who needs to know and understand what we're doing? Who can we persuade or engage by telling our story?

- **Document commitments:** Institutional shifts may be most apparent in mission statements, memoranda of understanding, negotiated contract language, student-family handbooks or staff guidance.

  Consider addressing questions such as: What policies and procedures best reflect our collective efforts? As our community continues to grow and shift, how can we orient and integrate new people and perspectives into these commitments without losing momentum?

Reflection

- To what extent do you agree that schools should be public health institutions?
- To what extent does your school community use or implement any of the models introduced in this chapter?

Recommended resource

"A Trauma Lens for Systems Change" by Patsy Carter and Andrea Blanch, **napnappartners.org/sites/default/files/Trauma%20Lens%20for%20systems%20change_Stanford%20Social%20Innovation%20Review_2019.pdf**

23 Champion the common good

CONTENT NOTE. This chapter is not likely to upset or trigger readers with references to specific forms of harm.

> *"Social justice involves our willingness to promote the common good of the communities to which we belong: literally, to will the good in and for others."*
>
> —Arthur James, Kristján Kristjánsson and Candace Vogler (Seeking the Good in Education Through a Positive Conception of Social Justice, 2020)

Social justice work in education is incomplete, partly because the term "social justice" has long focused on what we seek to prevent or thwart, rather than on what we actively agree to achieve (James, Kristjánsson, & Vogler, 2020). Furthermore, public education has not been a truly public good, but rather one subject to the same systems of oppression that plague other elements of our society (Justice, 2023). Unions are a key stakeholder in introducing and sustaining solidarity practices. This chapter reviews the labor movement's framework of bargaining for the common good and advocacy by workers-as-leaders to meet the promise of a just system of education.

Is public education good?

The status of public education in the U.S. is extremely dynamic; stakeholders differ on what should be a priority, the most effective methods and the appropriate impact of schools (Houston, 2025). While many assume that education is a shared good, education historians argue that education has disproportionately helped white families while harming people of color, constituting a racial good but not a common, or equitably shared, one (Justice, 2023; Ewing, 2025). Philosophers encourage trauma-informed educators to push past "negative justice," or what we do not want in education and to establish—or at least earnestly discuss—a positive conception of socially just education. Likewise, creating space for students to articulate their own visions and understandings of justice can also help them to develop a sense of their own lives and to prepare for full participation in the pursuit of the common good (James, Kristjánsson, & Vogler, 2020).

Workers as leaders

Authentic leadership expands the reach of educators' skills beyond traditional job descriptions, bringing their expertise and passion to new spaces. Leadership can look like mentoring colleagues, serving as department chair or multi-classroom coach, joining school building initiatives or advocating for more effective district-level policy or programming. Leadership programs are essential to sustainable and effective change efforts in schools and contribute to educator well-being (Vitucci & Brown, 2019; Proeschold-Bell, et al., 2021; Woo, LeTendre, Byun, & Schussler, 2022).

Since 2011, the AFT Teacher Leaders Program has helped prepare educators to identify, research and act on policy issues that impact the profession and student well-being. Each participating union site identifies and convenes a small group for a year to develop fellowship, professional learning communities and shared commitments to local action research for change. Program participants examine policy, conduct research, talk to policymakers and engage in public speaking. To conclude the year, Teacher Leaders explain their findings and share recommendations with policymakers at showcase events that catalyze further advocacy for policies and programs grounded in both strong evidence and their professional know-how (Vitucci & Brown, 2019; AFT, 2022). Leaders' participation also deepens connections to the union and broader community, undergirding support for public schools (Vitucci & Brown, 2019).

Bargain for the common good

Many educators are determined to make schooling a common good. Yet the pathways to doing so have felt fraught. Facing dwindling labor power, teacher unions across the nation have begun to rethink how to leverage one of their most fundamental tools: collective bargaining. In partnerships with worker centers, parents, indebted students and other beleaguered intersecting community groups, labor unions at the 2015 People's Congress set out to "establish a collective vision for social, racial and economic justice dismantle systems of racial discrimination and oppression; reclaim our democracy; reclaim our economy; reclaim our government [and] build the power of workers and workers' organizations" (McCartin, 2016).

Over the course of a decade, their efforts have grown into a national network of stakeholders who share power and campaign for investment in shared goals. Teacher unions have used this community organizing and contract negotiation approach to focus on what their community needs for human dignity and to win contract language and agreements on topics such as student homelessness and access to healthcare (Bargaining for the Common Good, 2025). The work is grounded in expansive yet concrete visions for public education.

Seven Key Elements of Bargaining for the Common Good (2020)

1. Expand the scope of bargaining beyond wages and benefits: Identify issues that resonate with members, partners and allies and that impact our communities. Put forth demands that address structural issues, not just symptoms of the problem.
2. Go on offense in a campaign by identifying, exposing and challenging the real villains, the financial and corporate actors who profit from and increasingly drive policies and actions.
3. Engage community allies as partners in issue development and the bargaining campaign: Bring in community partners on the ground floor and ask them what they need out of the bargaining campaign.
4. Center racial justice in demands: Campaign demands should address the role that employers play in creating and exacerbating structural racism in our communities.
5. Strengthen internal organizing, membership and member engagement: These campaigns must deeply engage the memberships of both unions and community organizations and there must be opportunities for deep relationship building and joint visioning between members of the different organizations.
6. Leverage capital in campaigns: We need to develop strategies that leverage the financial power of workers' pension funds and endowments to win common good demands.
7. The campaign doesn't end once the union settles its contract: Common good is about building long-term community-labor power, not about giving unions some good publicity during a contract fight. The boss doesn't automatically become a good actor once the contract is settled and the community's demands don't become any less important.

Reflections

- What forms of educator leadership are most visible in your school community?
- What are the primary challenges to education as a common good in your school community? Who is doing the strongest or most effective work on this?

Recommended resource

"Bargaining for the Common Good" from the Action Center on Race and the Economy, **bargainingforthecommongood.org**

24 Effectively engage families

CONTENT NOTE. This chapter is not likely to upset or trigger readers with references to specific forms of harm.

> *"Some people might view working with parents as separate from or supplemental to the daily work of teaching. But building relationships with children and caregivers should go hand in hand. [...] If teachers are unable to connect with caregivers, it is possible they simply have not yet discovered how."*
>
> —Edwards, et al. (Partnering with Families for Student Success: 24 Scenarios for Problem Solving with Parents, 2019)

A "good school" is one where diverse stakeholders experience belonging with a sense of community, trust, effective communication, goodwill and shared goals. Schools with powerful family engagement can (Stefanski, Valli, & Jacobson, 2016; Baker, Wise, Kelley, & Skiba, 2016; Jacques & Villegas, 2018; Ross, 2023):

- Better academic performance.
- Boost caregivers' knowledge of child development.
- Expand parents' confidence in teaching at home.
- Improve mutual attitudes, respect and trust between educators and caregivers.
- Increase attendance at school meetings.
- Increase student safety and school climate.
- Reduce disciplinary issues and extreme disciplinary tactics.

This chapter explores evidence-based practices to strengthen the bonds between key adults in children's lives—at home, at school and in the community.

Resource recipients ... or powerful parents?

Schools approach families with a continuum of programming perspectives that vary by assumptions about parent interest, capacity, barriers, strengths, as well as by goals and tactics (Stefanski, Valli, & Jacobson, 2016).

Serve: Schools raise awareness of select services and share information. Such service approaches tend to treat caregivers as learners, clients, beneficiaries and passive recipients of the school's expertise, resources and programs. These school-based efforts are often grounded in deficit-based beliefs and imply that parents need to be 'fixed' and that school professionals are best poised to identify and meet families' needs as institutional authorities (Ishimaru, 2017). These models also tend to assume the school is the default site for engagement and invite families to activities with parameters set by school staff.

Involve: Other models prioritize parents' involvement in school programs, sometimes as stakeholders in accomplishing goals set by school staff. This might look like inviting families into classrooms as volunteers or paid paraprofessionals or asking select caregivers to serve as liaisons and messengers, such as through faculty-family associations. Like service models, involvement programming is usually limited to the school site and typically generates low overall participation (Stefanski, Valli, & Jacobson, 2016).

Engage: Many researchers distinguish between 'involvement' or 'participation' and true family engagement. The distinction is about shared power. For example, at one point, Head Start defined family engagement as "goal-directed relationships between staff and families that are ongoing and culturally responsive; family and staff members share responsibility and mutually support what is best for children and families" (Stefanski, Valli, & Jacobson, 2016). Such programming requires schools to challenge typical hierarchies, improve effective communication and explore flexibility to achieve shared aims. Engaged parents act in roles with titles like "advisor," "board member" or "committee chair" and make decisions about things like program design and resource allocation.

Collaborate to transform: Family empowerment programs foster caregivers' leadership skills and contributions, such as to advocate, negotiate and represent the school beyond the building. They use words like "invest," "co-create" and "own" as they aim to overcome historical power gaps between educators and families. Empowerment models recognize parents as adults with their own unique strengths, assets, resources, expertise and agency (Stefanski, Valli, & Jacobson, 2016). Such equitable community–school collaborations necessitate:

- Systemic change goals
- Strategies that build capacity and relationships
- Caregivers from marginalized families in roles as experts and fellow educational leaders
- Educational change as a context-specific political process (Ishimaru, 2017)

Family empowerment changes *the school,* not just caregivers: "Relationships and a sense of shared experiences and concerns only go so far without parallel openings, shifts and capacity on the part of educators and school systems.

Rather, equitable collaboration suggests the need for shifts among educators and systems" (Ishimaru, 2017). It may look like funding family liaison positions to increase the languages spoken and cultures represented; sustaining evidence based family-faculty home visits; or parent leadership models so that participants become "recruiters, interpreters, workshop facilitators, trainers, curriculum developers, and even (formal) teachers" (Ishimaru, 2017).

Common barriers

Schools do not always achieve their goals to engage families. Fewer than 40 percent of educators feel adequately prepared to do so (Peltier, et al., 2025). Educators commonly cite parents' previous negative experiences with school, logistical barriers and disinterest as sticking points (Baker, Wise, Kelley, & Skiba, 2016).

On the other hand, when asked, "What does not work in engaging families?" parents often name educators' judgmental attitudes (Kelty & Wakabayashi, 2020). For example, parents who experience unwelcoming front office staff often decide against interacting with other school personnel (Siegel, et al., 2018). Such negative interactions are linked to feelings of inadequacy and inferiority with school staff (Baker, Wise, Kelley, & Skiba, 2016). Furthermore, caregivers cite:

- Alienating school bureaucracy, such as complicated paperwork and duplicate procedures
- Poor timing of communication from schools that does not allow them to plan to shift routines or life logistics
- Logistical and practical constraints such as transportation issues, work schedules, need for childcare and need to feed, especially when they have multiple children
- Language and cultural barriers that push parents to both translate or code-switch and process information, often without support
- Staff failures to effectively interrupt bullying or show grief-sensitivity (Baker, Wise, Kelley, & Skiba, 2016; Siegel, et al., 2018)

Effective family engagement

Trauma-informed educators overcome barriers and connect with families by practicing key skills (Peltier, et al., 2025; National Association of Family, School, and Community Engagement, 2022; Ball, Skrzypek, & Lynch, 2020; Siegel, et al., 2018; Kelty & Wakabayashi, 2020; Edwards, et al., 2019; Ross, 2023):

- **Respect, honor and value families:** Center interactions around safety, choices, collaboration, trustworthiness and empowerment; withhold judgment of caregivers and assumptions about motivations, capacity or desire, especially when these were not communicated.

- **Embrace equity:** Ask about the family's goals and needs; tailor immediate and ongoing support; practice cognitive flexibility, perspective taking and humility to combat bias and contextualize specific challenges, which may include illiteracy, second language fluency or homelessness.
- **Build trusting and reciprocal relationships with families:** Listen, be flexible, genuine and honest; communicate frequently; identify caregiver strengths.
- **Co-construct learning opportunities with families:** Examine and respect a family's knowledge and strengths as resources; make a plan for two-way communication; follow through and revisit shared goals.
- **Link family engagement to learning and development:** Give families the tools to actively engage in their child's education; conduct outreach for students at every developmental stage.
- **Take part in lifelong learning:** Seek professional development and training opportunities to build confidence and capacity; practice critical reflection to propel the field and yourself.
- **Advocate for system change:** Shift the idea of parent involvement and family engagement away from the school-as-site and toward collaboration for authentic student growth; identify opportunities to support family empowerment with new policy and practice.

Furthermore, schools as institutions can flexibly schedule events with attention to work schedules, mealtimes and students' siblings; iteratively communicate updates as opportunities approach, in appropriate languages and through a variety of channels; streamline requirements for parents to be at school, including during class time; treat events that occur outside of a school building, such as at the library or local recreation center, as constructive family engagement with their children's education; and prepare educators to address diverse cultural, class and experiential backgrounds through deliberate training (Baker, Wise, Kelley, & Skiba, 2016).

Home Visits

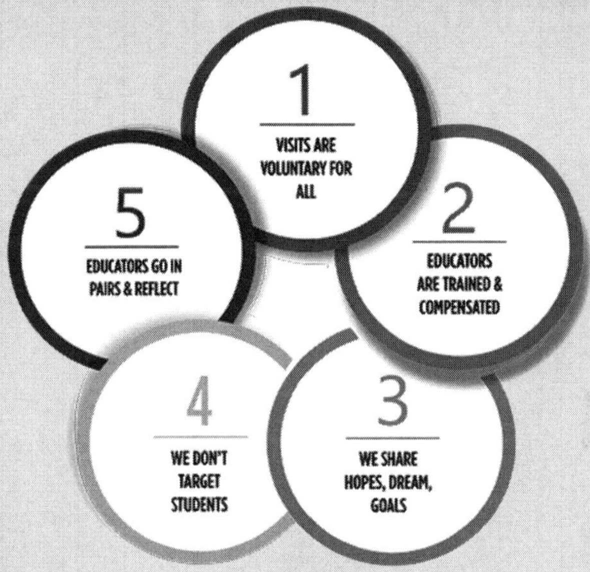

The Five Non-Negotiables of Parent Teacher Home Visits include voluntary participation, training and compensation for educators, a strengths-based approach that eschews shame and educators who pair to both visit and reflect (Parent Teacher Home Visits, 2025).

Nearly 30 years ago, parents used community organizing principles to build trust and accountability with educators and interrupt cycles of blame. They innovated a home visit, a voluntary meeting between adults as equals, away from any institutional setting and focused on jointly hearing each other's answers to the question, "What are your hopes and dreams for this child?" Refined and then piloted by a teacher union, a parent organizing group and the local school district, the project inspired a new nonprofit with a footprint far beyond its Sacramento roots. More than 50,000 trained educators have made over 300,000 home visits in 30 states (Parent Teacher Home Visits Project, 2023).

Reflections

- Which family programming model best reflects your school community? How could your school better engage or empower families?
- This chapter lists seven skills for effective family engagement. How many of them have been part of your training to date?

Recommended resource

"The Case for Strong Family and Community Engagement in Schools" by Elizabeth M. Ross, **gse.harvard.edu/ideas/usable-knowledge/23/03/case-strong-family-and-community-engagement-schools**

25 Institutionalize mandated support

CONTENT NOTE. This chapter includes ideas related to abuse, child maltreatment, family separation and neglect.

> *"Understanding that harm originates from situations dominated by stress, scarcity, and oppression, one way to prevent violence is to make sure that people have support to get the things they need. We must also create a culture that enables people to actually take accountability for violence and harm."*
>
> —Mariame Kaba and Kelly Hayes (The Sentencing of Larry Nassar Was Not 'Transformative Justice.' Here's Why., 2021)

Child protection is not just a government agency, but a collective responsibility—and schools are a critical component of effective child maltreatment prevention (Malvaso, Pilkington, Montgomerie, Delfabbro, & Lynch, 2020; Institute to Transform Child Protection, 2025). This chapter builds on the critical analysis of mandatory reporting and systemic outcomes in "Reduce the risk of abuse." We examine school- and district-level opportunities to implement the invitations embedded in mandated support.

JMACforFamilies coined the term "mandated support" to prioritize intact families and reduce harm. Under this umbrella, advocates work to:

- Elevate prevention over lagging intervention.
- Eliminate unnecessary reporting to government agencies.
- Prioritize compassionate curiosity and creativity over compliance grounded in fear or punishment.
- Support, rather than separate, families.

Uphold due process

Due process is a civil right and essential in the labor movement. This big idea includes the right to have fair, reasonable and established rules govern proceedings, especially when facing punishment for possible wrongdoing. Yet due process is often abandoned when addressing maltreatment (Brennan, 2020;

Richards & Fromknecht, 2024). Trauma-informed schools uphold due process for all stakeholders.

Tell families their rights

The Fourth Amendment to the Constitution protects against unreasonable search and seizure. In practice, the government usually must show that it has good reason to intrude into private lives, such as through a warrant, court order or proof of immediate danger. CPS routinely skips this step, instead coercing families to comply with invasive investigations and interventions by misrepresenting rights and responsibilities (Sciacca, 2023; Hager, 2022; L.B. v City of New York, Slip Copy, 2025).

Trauma-informed schools can include plain "Know Your Rights" messaging about mandatory reporting and CPS in communication to families, such as through a handbook. More substantively, schools can establish and adhere to processes that require CPS' due diligence. When asked to contribute to or participate in active investigations of maltreatment, schools can require a court order and subject CPS documentation to review by legal counsel. Such steps to establish equal footing for families in child welfare investigations encourage CPS to be more transparent, inspire families to be more forthcoming and ultimately improve child safety outcomes (Trivedi S., 2025).

Default to support—for the education workforce

Educators are much more likely to interact with CPS as mandatory reporters than as subjects of investigation. However, in rare instances, schools, districts and unions have important opportunities to uphold due process for the workforce, as well. First, educators are almost never charged with failure to report (Woodnick & Ranney, 2022; M. Itzkowitz, personal communication, February 20, 2025). When cases are pursued, educators' judgment is typically held against the standard of "reasonable suspicion" (William, 2009; Skulina, 2010; McDonald, 2013; People v. Davis, 2005; Meier v. Salem-Keizer School District, 2017; Roe v. Hesperia Unified School District, 2022). Second, each year a small group of educators are the subject of reports to CPS. Educators facing such charges encounter serious professional consequences, whether the allegations relate to the workplace—even when the report was not verified (M. Lombreglia, L. Bossing, and J. McMillan, personal communication).

For both types of challenges, unions and districts can assure fair proceedings by streamlining access to competent representation for educators. Such a commitment could build on existing statutory language:

> *In cases in which an employee subject to the state mandatory reporting law acts in good faith and without negligence in their reporting duty, and if the employee's judgment as to what constitutes reasonable cause to believe that a child has suffered abuse or neglect*

is being challenged, the District and union shall equally share costs to provide for the legal defense of the employee (Washington State Legislature, 2024).

Create cultures of compassion

School-level policy and culture strongly influence educator reporting behaviors (Prax, Nobody Wins, 2025). Districts and unions are responsible for developing school cultures where child protection is understood as a collective responsibility and:

- Educators are prepared to strengthen protective connections and warmly refer to supports.
- Consultation, compassion, curiosity and collaboration are the defaults when facing complexity.
- Reporting to CPS is a last resort and undertaken with robust review of ethical and legal duties (Institute to Transform Child Protection, 2025).

Prepare educators to respond, not just react

Most workforce training on child maltreatment focuses on how to report and boosts confidence (McTavish, et al., 2017; Brown, Bowyer, & Walsh, 2024; Pietrantoni, Chitiyo, Chitiyo, Peña, & Fernandez, 2023). But confidence does not predict quality and the evidence is "low to very low" that training improves outcomes, including accuracy (Walsh, et al., 2022; Brown, Bowyer, & Walsh, 2024). Furthermore, most training fails to prepare educators to face real-world issues or extend support at critical moments (Institute to Transform Child Protection, 2025). Educators need training on relevant knowledge and skills that prepare them to do more than just report, but to reflect and respond with curiosity and creativity. Robust professional learning should address objectives such as:

- Read and analyze the state code related to mandatory reporting.
- Critically reflect on ability, class, cultural, linguistic, racial and other biases, including in their own observations and assessments.
- Leverage ethical frameworks to grapple with realistic ethical dilemmas and address moral injury.
- Evaluate the likelihood of CPS substantiation and service delivery, as well as further harm.
- Map local supports and alternatives to CPS.
- Practice strategies for direct dialogue with families, including with reluctant caregivers facing layered life challenges.

Make it easy to support

Concrete, material support to families consistently reduces child maltreatment (Cusick, et al., 2024; Pac, et al., 2023). In addition to effective anti-poverty programming to meet material needs, families at risk of CPS engagement benefit from connections to programs and providers that address adult substance use, mental illness and high-quality childcare (Palmer, Font, Eastman, Guo, & Putnam-Hornstein, 2024). Whole-school, whole-child, whole-community initiatives are therefore a powerful way to prevent child maltreatment. Systemic interventions to address child maltreatment are most impactful when they:

- Leverage democratic collaboration between school personnel and community.
- Combine formal and informal supports.
- Engage both leaders, such as superintendents and school boards, as well as end-users, such as caregivers (Lo & Cho, 2021).

Reflections

- Many of the interventions outlined in this chapter are intimately linked to others in the book, including family engagement, whole-school, whole-child and whole-community (WSCC) initiatives and the common good. How can you leverage existing efforts to make progress toward mandated support?
- "Reduce the risk of abuse" outlines that fear, ambiguity, poverty and bias are some of the core reasons that 'child protection' so often achieves harm. To what extent do these factors reflect challenges you anticipate in institutionalizing mandated support? How can you collaborate and plan to address those challenges?

Recommended resource

"Mandated Support in Education: Protecting Children by Assisting Families" by Chelsea Prax, **bit.ly/3DiKZFK**

Acknowledgments

For over a decade, I have had the honor of developing professional learning content and training experiences for educators and AFT members. The journey to this iteration of the student trauma course—including this book—reflects many people's generous and thoughtful engagement.

Shannon Lederer's kind mentorship and stirring analysis was a smiling, open door into the labor movement. Darryl Alexander offered me the first professional opportunity to weave together training in public health with experiences in the classroom—and trusted me to carry sufficient verve into unfamiliar spaces to make myself heard.

Marla Ucelli-Kashyap and Giselle Lundy-Ponce greenlight so many of my hare-brained schemes; I am grateful for the resulting chances to grow in new directions. Lisa Dickinson reinvigorated AFT's connection to Trinity College; that institutional partnership is a quiet reminder to model consistency and quality, which I endeavored to achieve here.

Lonna Davis, Brian O'Connor, Tien Ung and the Futures Without Violence crew take my questions seriously, nudge me forward and earnestly partner. You have so gently and fiercely changed my mind and my life; I hope you see my admiration here.

Joyce McMillan and Kelley Fong welcomed me early with open arms into an entirely different way of applying what I know of public health, trauma-informed practices and careful school health interventions. I am grateful to walk with titans toward new horizons.

Dr. Kimberly Harmon Welch affirmed my hard work and mirrored it back to me with her own. In addition to being my brilliant colleague, Dr. Lisa Thomas is an unspeakably good friend who listens with care whether I bring frustration or confusion or triumph.

Melanie Boyer is direct and cutting and kind and so deliciously funny while making sure my writing is good enough. Jen Dubin brought aplomb to a task I find absolutely loathsome. Amy Darling is thorough and creative, a magical combination necessary to turn a looong document into a real-deal book.

A small dream team conspires with me to transform research into sustainable skills and institutional change: The eight letters in "thank you" drown in my gratitude. Jim has full custody of his inner child and takes me on rollercoasters with his imagination, ambition and follow-through. Melissa is a study in hard-won self-love. She radiates contagious calm (that furious churning never breaks the surface) and reminds me to take the most complicated things one step at a time. Kim teaches me to set intentions beyond my fingertips, to deliberately cultivate collective emotional energy. Her kindness is legendary and a purposeful legacy. It is a gift to laugh with you all, despite [glances around] ... nuns and puppies!

Index

References

Advancement Project, AFT, NEA & National Opportunity to Learn Campaign. (2014). *Restorative practices: Fostering healthy relationships & promoting positive discipline in schools.* advancementproject.org/resources/restorative-practices-fostering-healthy-relationships-promoting-positive-discipline-in-schools/

AFT. (2021, February 1). *A century of progress* [Video]. YouTube. youtube.com/watch?v=vYKorR9yYAU

AFT. (2015). *Educator quality of work life: Executive summary.*

AFT. (2017). *Educator quality of work life: Executive summary.* bit.ly/2zyQVID

AFT. (2020). *Living wage campaign toolkit.* aft.org/sites/default/files/media/documents/2022/Living%20Wage%20Toolkit%20Interactive.pdf

AFT. (2022). *Making connections, building capacity: How AFT supports our members and our profession through educational issues.* aft.org/reports/making-connections-building-capacity

AFT & Educators Thriving. (2023). *Beyond burnout: A roadmap to improve educator well-being.* aft.org/sites/default/files/media/documents/2023/Beyond_Burnout_A_Roadmap_to_Improve_Educator_Wellbeing.pdf

AFT & New York Life Foundation. (2020). *New York Life Foundation and American Federation of Teachers grief in school survey: Key findings and topline results.* newyorklife.com/assets/foundation/docs/pdfs/key-findings-and-topline.pdf

Allen, S. (2018). *The science of gratitude.* Greater Good Science Center. ggsc.berkeley.edu/images/uploads/GGSC-JTF_White_Paper-Gratitude-FINAL.pdf

All4Ed. (2019). *Ten things to know about trauma and learning.* all4ed.org/blog/ten-things-to-know-about-trauma-and-learning/

Au, W., & Hagopian, J. (2018). How one elementary school sparked a citywide movement to make Black students' lives matter. In D. Watson, J. Hagopian, & W. Au (Eds.), *Teaching for Black lives* (pp. 22–31). Rethinking Schools.

Bach, D., Groesbeck, G., Stapleton, P., Sims, R., Blickheuser, K., & Church, D. (2019). Clinical EFT (Emotional Freedom Techniques) improves multiple physiological markers of health. *Journal of Evidence-Based Integrative Medicine, 24.* doi:10.1177/2515690X18823691

Baker, C. N., Augenstern, J. M., Moberg, S. A., Robey, N., & Saybe, M. C. (2020). Developing school staff buy-in for trauma-informed schools. In E. Rossen (Ed.), *Supporting and educating traumatized students: A guide for school-based professionals* (pp. 359–371). Oxford University Press.

Baker, T. L., Wise, J., Kelley, G., & Skiba, R. J. (2016). Identifying barriers: Creating solutions to improve family engagement. *School Community Journal, 26*(2), 163–184. adi.org/journal/2016fw/BakerEtAlFall2016.pdf

Ball, A., Skrzypek, C., & Lynch, M. (2020). The family engagement practice framework: A comprehensive framework developed from the voices of school-based practitioners. *Family Relations Interdisciplinary Journal of Applied Family Science, 70*(4), 1190–1205. doi:10.1111/fare.12513

Bargaining for the Common Good. (2020). *Key elements of bargaining for the common good campaigns.* bargainingforthecommongood.org/wp-content/uploads/2020/04/BCG-Seven-Elements.pdf

Bargaining for the Common Good. (2025). *Network updates.* bargainingforthecommongood.org

Barrett, M. S. (n.d.). *Ethical issues and decision-making in the treatment of trauma.* DHSS Division of Substance Abuse and Mental Health. dhss.delaware.gov/dsamh/files/si2013_ethicalissuesandtrauma.pdf

Barth, R., Johnson-Reid, M., Greeson, J., Drake, B., Berrick, J., Garcia, A., Shaw, T., & Gyourko, J. (2020). Outcomes following child welfare services: What are they and do they differ for Black children? *Journal of Public Child Welfare, 14*(5), 477–499. doi: 10.1080/15548732.2020.1814541

Bass, R., Imad, M., Powers, K., Njaka, I., Peacock, D., Barranco, K., & Bryant, K. (2023). *Cycles of trauma and the journey to wellbeing: A framework for trauma-informed practices and positive social change.* The Being and Transforming Think Tank. static1.squarespace.com/static/651d64da5cf17441ae31ba8d/t/65e85189b567545b395de867/1709724044054/ExecSummary_CyclesOfTrauma.pdf

Baughman, C., Coles, T., Feinberg, J., & Newton, H. (2021). The surveillance tentacles of the child welfare system. *Columbia Journal of Race and Law, 11*(3), 501–532. journals.library.columbia.edu/index.php/cjrl/article/view/8743/4502

Berger, E. (2019). Multi-tiered approaches to trauma-informed care in schools: A systematic review. *School Mental Health, 11*, 650–664. doi:10.1007/s12310-019-09326-0

Bernstein, M., & Pfefferbaum, B. (2018). Posttraumatic growth as a response to natural disasters in children and adolescents. *Current Psychiatry Reports, 20*(5), 37. doi:10.1007/s11920-018-0900-4

Bernadel, S., Fiddiman, B., Jackson, B., Raben, C., Alexandre, E., Del Miami, M., Santon, S., Tucker, L., Tucker, M., Clark, T., Girl Power Rocks, Overtown Youth Center, & Power, U.. (2024). *Keep her safe: Centering Black girls in school safety.* National Women's Law Center. nwlc.org/resource/keep-her-safe-centering-black-girls-in-school-safety/#

Bistricky, S., Jong, L., Lai, B., Gallagher, M., Kanenberg, H., Elkins, S., Harper, K.S., & Short, M. (2019, October). Surviving the storm: Avoidant coping, helping behavior, resilience and affective symptoms around a major hurricane-flood. *Journal of Affective Disorders, 257*, 297–306. doi:10.1016/j.jad.2019.07.044

Black, D. (2022). *Don't cry for me.* Hanover Square Press.

Blake, J. J., & Epstein, R. (2019). *Listening to Black women and girls: Lived experiences of adultification bias.* Georgetown Center on Law and Poverty. chrome-extension://efaidnbmnnnibpcajpcglclefindmkaj/https://www.law.georgetown.edu/poverty-inequality-center/wp-content/uploads/sites/14/2019/05/Listening-to-Black-Women-and-Girls.pdf

Blaustein, M. E., & Kinniburgh, K. M. (2019). *Treating traumatic stress in children and adolescents: How to foster resilience through attachment, self-regulation, and competency.* Guilford Press.

Bloodworth, M. R., & Horner, A. C. (2019). *Return on investment of a community school coordinator: A case study.* Albuquerque: Apex and ABC Community School Partnership. communityschools.org/wp-content/uploads/sites/2/2020/11/ROI_Coordinator.pdf

Boltz, L. O., Henriksen, D., Mishra, P., & Deep-Play Research Group, M. S. (2015). Rethinking technology & creativity in the 21st century: Empathy through gaming—perspective taking in a complex world. *TechTrends, 59*(6), 3–6. danah-henriksen.com/wp-content/uploads/2015/11/techtrends-empathy.pdf

Bor, J., Venkataramani, A. S., Williams, D. R., & Tsai, A. C. (2018, July). Police killings and their spillover effects on the mental health of Black Americans: A population-based, quasi-experimental study. *The Lancet, 392*(10144), 302–310. doi:10.1016/S0140-6736(18)31130-9

Bowman, D., & Popp, P. A. (2020). Students experiencing homelessness. In E. Rossen (Ed.), *Supporting and educating traumatized students: A guide for school-based professionals* (pp. 125–145). Oxford University Press.

Bren, S. (Host). (2024, March 19). Using presence as the antidote to trauma: How we begin to break cycles with Dr. Jacob Ham [Audio podcast episode]. In *Securely Attached.* drsarahbren.com/186-using-presence-as-the-antidote-to-trauma-how-we-begin-to-break-cycles-with-dr-jacob-ham/

Brennan, J. (2020). Emergency removals without a court order: Using the language of emergency to duck due process. *Journal of Law and Policy, 29*(1). brooklynworks.brooklaw.edu/jlp/vol29/iss1/3

Brunzell, T., Stokes, H., & Waters, L. (2016). Trauma-informed flexible learning: Classrooms that strengthen regulatory abilities. *International Journal of Child, Youth and Family Studies, 7*(2), 218–239. doi:10.18357/ijcyfs72201615719

Brunzell, T., Stokes, H., & Waters, L. (2019). Shifting teacher practice in trauma-affected classrooms: Practice pedagogy strategies within a trauma-informed positive education model. *School Mental Health, 11*, 600–614. doi.org/10.1007/s12310-018-09308-8

Brown, M., Bowyer, J., & Walsh, K. (2024). School counsellors' reporting child maltreatment: A rapid review of empirical evidence. *Australian Psychologists and Counsellors in Schools, 34*(3). doi.org/10.1177/20556365241262552

Brunzell, T., Waters, L., & Stokes, H. (2015). Teaching with strengths in trauma-affected students: A new approach to healing and growth in the classroom. *American Journal of Orthopsychiatry, 85*(1), 3–9. doi:10.1037/ort0000048

Burns, M., Landry, L., Mills, D., Carlson, N., Blueford, J. M., & Talmi, A. (2023, March 29). COVID-19 pandemic's disproportionate impact on childhood bereavement for youth of color: Reflections and recommendations. *Frontiers in Pediatrics, 11*, 1–8. doi:10.3389/fped.2023.1063449

Calderon de la Barca, L., Milligan, K., & Kania, J. (2024, February 12). Healing systems. *Stanford Social Innovation Review.* ssir.org/articles/entry/healing-trauma-systems

Carlton, M. P. (2017). *Summary of school safety statistics.* National Institute of Justice. files.eric.ed.gov/fulltext/ED575741.pdf

Carter, P., & Blanch, A. (2019). A trauma lens for systems change. *Stanford Social Innovation Review*, 48–54. napnappartners.org/sites/default/files/Trauma%20Lens%20for%20systems%20change_Stanford%20Social%20Innovation%20Review_2019.pdf

The Center for Health and Healthcare in Schools. (2018). *Partner build grow: An action guide for sustaining child development and prevention approaches.* actionguide.healthinschools.org

Center on the Developing Child. (2015). In brief: What is resilience? [Video]. YouTube. youtube.com/watch?v=cqO7YoMsccU&

Centers for Disease Control and Prevention. (2018, September 25). *Preventing adverse childhood experiences (ACEs) online training module 2 Lesson 1: Video 3 of 3 AD* [Video]. YouTube. youtube.com/watch?v=-1c2X5T7frw

Centers for Disease Control and Prevention. (2019, November). Adverse childhood experiences (ACEs): Preventing early trauma to improve adult health. *Vital Signs*. cdc.gov/vitalsigns/aces/pdf/vs-1105-aces-H.pdf

Centers for Disease Control and Prevention. (2021, April 6). *About the CDC-Kaiser ACE Study.* cdc.gov/violenceprevention/aces/about.html

Centers for Disease Control and Prevention. (2022). Adolescent behaviors and experiences survey—United States, January–June 2021. *Morbidity and Mortality Weekly Report, 71*(3), Supplement. U.S. Department of Health and Human Services. cdc.gov/mmwr/volumes/71/su/pdfs/su7103a1-a5-H.pdf

Centers for Disease Control and Prevention. (2024). *Youth risk behavior survey data summary & trends report: 2013–2023.* U.S. Department of Health and Human Services. cdc.gov/yrbs/dstr/index.html

Childhood Bereavement Estimation Model. (2021). Childhood bereavement: Race and ethnicity. Judi's House / JAG Institute. Retrieved from https://judishouse.org/research-tools/cbem/cbem-key-topics/cbem-race-and-ethnicity/cbem-race-ethnicity-reports/

Childhood Bereavement Estimation Model. (2023). *2023 CBEM pandemic impact report.* Judi's House / JAG Institute. judishouse.org/research-tools/cbem/cbem-key-topics/pandemic-impact/2023-cbem-pandemic-impact-report/

Childhood Bereavement Estimation Model. (2024). *CBEM national report 2024.* Judi's House / JAG Institute. judishouse.org/research-tools/cbem

Children's Bureau. (2024). *Child maltreatment 2022.* U. S. Department of Health and Human Services, Administration for Children and Families. acf.hhs.gov/cb/data-research/child-maltreatment

Church, D., Stapleton, P., Yang, A., & Gallo, F. (2018). Is tapping on acupuncture points an active ingredient in emotional freedom techniques? A systematic review and meta-analysis of comparative studies. *The Journal of Nervous and Mental Disease, 206*(10), 783–793. researchgate.net/profile/Dawson-Church/publication/328002243_Is_Tapping_on_Acupuncture_Points_an_Active_Ingredient_in_Emotional_Freedom_Techniques_A_Systematic_Review_and_Meta-analysis_of_Comparative_Studies/links/5c575870299bf12be3fa8577/Is-T

Civitillo, S., Mayer, A.-M., & Jugert, P. (2023). A systematic review and meta-analysis of the associations between perceived teacher-based racial–ethnic discrimination and student well-being and academic outcomes. *Journal of Educational Psychology 116*(5), 719–741. doi:10.1037/edu0000818

Clarren, R. (2023). *The cost of free land: Jews, Lakota, and an American inheritance.* Penguin Random House.

Cook, E., & Black, P. (2020). Effective implementation and evaluation of trauma-informed schools. In E. Rossen (Ed.), *Supporting and educating traumatized students: A guide for school-based personnel* (pp. 373–395). Oxford University Press.

Cooper, M., & Thesing, E. (Hosts). (2023, April 7). We keep us safe [Audio podcast episode]. In Dancing on Desks. podcasters.spotify.com/pod/show/dancingondesks/episodes/Season-2--Episode-5--We-Keep-Us-Safe-e1vqqor

Crittenden, P. M., & Spieker, S. (2023). The effects of separation from parents on children. In D. Kelly (Ed.), *Understanding child abuse and neglect: Research and implications.*doi: 10.5772/intechopen.1002940

Cuartas, J., Salazar, A., Backhaus, S., Little, M. T., McCoy, D., Yoshikawa, H., Bass, M., Metheny, N., & Knaul, F. (2024). Strategies to prevent violence against children in the home: A systematic review of reviews. *Trauma, Violence, & Abuse, 25*(4), 3419–3433. doi:10.1177/15248380241247018

Cummings, K. P., Addante, S., Swindell, J., & Meadan, H. (2017). Creating supportive environments for children who have had exposure to traumatic events. *Journal of Child and Family Studies, 26*, 2728–2741. doi:10.1007/s10826-017-0774-9

Curren, R. (2020). Punishment and motivation in a just school community. *Theory and Research in*

Education, 18(1), 117–133. doi:10.1177/1477878520916089

Cusick, G., Gaul-Stout, J., Kakuyama-Villaber, R., Wilks, O., Grewal-Kök, Y., & Anderson, C. (2024). A systematic review of economic and concrete support to prevent child maltreatment. *Societies, 14*(9), 173. doi:10.3390/soc14090173

Darawsheh, S., Asha, I., AbuSaif, R., Alhejoj, A., & Khasawneh, M. (2023). An outline of the professional quality of teachers who teach children with special needs. *Journal of Education and e-Learning Research, 10*(3), 358–363. files.eric.ed.gov/fulltext/EJ1408079.pdf

Darling-Hammond, L., Flook, L., Cook-Harvey, C., Barron, B., & Osher, D. (2019). Implications for the educational practice of the science of learning and development. *Applied Developmental Science, 24*(2), 97–140. doi:10.1080/10888691.2018.1537791

Darling-Hammond, S. (2023). *Fostering belonging, transforming schools: The impact of restorative practices.* Learning Policy Institute. learningpolicyinstitute.org/product/impact-restorative-practices-report

Day, A. G., Baroni, B., Somers, C., Shier, J., Zammit, M., Crosby, S., Yoon, J., Pennefather, M., & Hong, J. S. (2017). Trauma and triggers: Students' perspectives on enhancing the classroom experiences at an alternative residential treatment school. *Children and Schools, 39*(4), 227–337. academia.edu/download/54989705/traumas_and_triggers.pdf

DeAngelis, T. (2019). The legacy of trauma. *Monitor on Psychology, 50*(2), 36. apa.org/monitor/2019/02/legacy-trauma

Densen, A., Lansworth, T., & Siegel, L. (2012, December 10). *Groundbreaking survey of educators shows overwhelming interest in helping grieving students—And strong demand for training, more support.* AFT and New York Life Foundation. aft.org/sites/default/files/media/2015/release_bereavement121012.pdf

DePanfilis, D. (2018). *Child protective services: A guide for caseworkers.* U.S. Children's Bureau. resourcecentre.savethechildren.net/document/child-protective-services-guide-caseworkers-2018

DeStigter, L. F. (2018). *Healthy school, healthy staff, healthy students: A guide to improving school employee wellness.* National Association of Chronic Disease Directors. https://stacks.cdc.gov/view/cdc/61302

Detlaff, A., Weber, K., Pendleton, M., Boyd, R., Bettencourt, B., & Burton, L. (2020). It is not a broken system, it is a system that needs to be broken: The upEND movement to abolish the child welfare system. *Journal of Public Child Welfare, 14*(5), 500–517. tandfonline.com/doi/full/10.1080/15548732.2020.1814542

Doe, H., Osborne, C., Huffman, J., Craig, S., & Shero, M. (2025). Home visiting and child welfare involvement: A matched comparison group study. *Child Maltreatment, 30*(2), 1–12. doi:10.1177/10775595241268227

Dolezal, L., & Gibson, M. (2022). Beyond a trauma-informed approach and towards shame-sensitive practice. *Humanities and Social Science Communications, 9*, 214. doi:10.1057/s41599-022-01227-z

Dombo, E. A., & Sabatino, C. A. (2019). Trauma care in schools. *American Educator*, 18–21. aft.org/ae/summer2019/dombo_sabatino

Drulis, C., Matz, T., Samuelson, C., & Cozolino, L. (2021, December). Restoring relationships, healing trauma, and creating securely attached classrooms. *Journal of Higher Education Theory and Practice, 21*(13). articlegateway.com/index.php/JHETP/article/view/4797

Dunbar, A. S., Zeytinoglu, S., & Leerkes, E. M. (2022). When is parental suppression of Black children's negative emotions adaptive? The role of preparation for racial bias and children's resting cardiac vagal tone. *Research on Child and Adolescent Psychopathology, 50*(2), 163–176. doi:10.1007/s10802-021-00779-z

Dunning, D., Tudor, K., Radley, L., Dalrymple, N., Funk, J., Vainre, M., . . . Dalgleish, T. (2022). Do mindfulness-based programmes improve the cognitive skills, behaviour and mental health of children and adolescents? An updated meta-analysis of randomised controlled trials. *Evidence-Based Mental Health.* doi:10.1136/ebmental-2022-300464

Editors of Rethinking Schools. (2019). Little kids, big ideas: Teaching social issues and global conflicts with young children. In L. Christensen, S. Karp, B. Peterson, & M. Yonamine (Eds.), *The new teacher book: Finding purpose, balance, and hope during your first years in the classroom* (pp. 298–301). Rethinking Schools.

Education Civil Rights Alliance & AFT. (2020). *Police in schools: A background paper.* youthlaw.org/resources/police-schools-background-paper

Educator Policy Innovation Center. (2017). *From exclusionary to restorative: An intentional, trauma-sensitive approach to interrupting racial disparities, reducing violence, strengthening communities, and accelerating student learning.* Education Minnesota. educationminnesota.org/wp-content/uploads/2021/08/EPIC-student-discipline-report.pdf

Edwards, B. (2021, October 23). The man behind unconditional positive regard. *Psychology Today.* psychologytoday.com/intl/blog/progress-notes/202110/the-man-behind-unconditional-positive-regard

Edwards, P. A., Spiro, R. J., Domke, L. M., Castle, A. M., White, K. L., Peltier, M. R., & Donohue, T. H. (2019). *Partnering with families for student success: 24 scenarios for problem solving with parents.* Teachers College Press.

Eklund, K., Koriakin, T. A., Chafouleas, S. M., & Dodge, S. C. (2020). Trauma screening and assessment. In E. Rossen (Ed.), *Supporting and Educating Traumatized Students: A Guide for School-Based Professionals* (pp. 325–341). Oxford University Press.

Ellis, B. J., Abrams, L. S., Masten, A. S., Sternberg, R. J., Tottenham, N., & Frankenhuis, W. E. (2020). Hidden talents in harsh environments. *Development and Psychopathology, 34*(1), 95–113. doi:10.1017/S0954579420000887

Evangelist, M., Thomas, M., & Waldfogel, J. (2023). Child protective services contact and youth outcomes. *Child Abuse & Neglect, 136*(105994). doi: 10.1016/j.chiabu.2022.105994

Evans, K., & Vaandering, D. (2016). *The little book of restorative justice in education: Fostering responsibility, healing, and hope in schools.* Good Books.

Ewing, E. L. (2025). *Original sins: The miseducation of Black and Native children and the construction of American racism.* One World.

Fisher, J. (1999). The work of stabilization in trauma treatment. *The Trauma Center Lecture Series.* HRI Hospital. smchealth.org/sites/main/files/file-attachments/tic_stabilize.pdf

Fong, K. (2023). *Investigating families: Motherhood in the shadow of child protective services.* Princeton University Press.

Foo, S. (2022). *What my bones know: A memoir of healing from complex trauma.* Ballantine Books.

Ford, J. D., King, N., Galappaththi, E. K. , Pearce, T., McDowell, G., & Harper, S. L. (2020). The resilience of Indigenous peoples to environmental change. *One Earth, 2*(6), 532–543. doi:https://doi.org/10.1016/j.oneear.2020.05.014

Forde, A. T., Crookes, D. M., Suglia, S. F., & Demmer, R. T. (2019). The weathering hypothesis as an explanation for racial disparities in health: A systematic review. *Annals of Epidemiology, 33*, 1–18.e3. doi:https://doi.org/10.1016/j.annepidem.2019.02.011

Fortin, K., Kwon, S., & Pierce, M. (2016). Characteristics of children reported to child protective services for medical neglect. *Hospital Pediatrics, 6*(4), 204–210. doi:10.1542/hpeds.2015-0151

Fraguas, D., Diaz-Caneja, C. M., Ayora, M., Durán-Cutilla, M., Abregú-Crespo, R., Ezquiaga-Bravo, I., Martín-Babarro, J., & Arango, C. (2021). Assessment of school anti-bullying interventions. *JAMA Pediatrics, 175*(1), 44–55. doi:10.1001/jamapediatrics.2020.3541

Frederickson, B. L. (2004, September 29). The broaden-and-build theory of positive emotions. *Philosophical Transactions of the Royal Society: Biological Sciences, 359*(1449), 1367–1378. doi:10.1098/rstb.2004.1512

Friere, P. (2007). *Pedagogy of the oppressed* (30th anniversary ed.). Continuuum.

Fronius, T., Darling-Hammond, S., Persson, H., Guckenberg, S., Hurley, N., & Petrosino, A. (2019). *Restorative justice in U.S. schools.* WestEd. files.eric.ed.gov/fulltext/ED595733.pdf

Futures Without Violence. (2025). *Gestures that can heal.* changingmindsnow.org/gestures

Garcia Mathewson, T. (2022, June 6). *'State-sanctioned violence:' Inside one of the thousands of schools that still paddle students.* The Hechinger Report. hechingerreport.org/state-sanctioned-violence-inside-one-of-the-thousands-of-schools-that-still-paddles-students/

Gendre, E., Soubelet, A., & Callahan, S. (2025). Trajectories of posttraumatic growth identified from person-centered analyses: A systematic review. *European Journal of Trauma & Dissociation, 9*(1), 100485. doi:10.1016/j.ejtd.2024.100485

Gilligan, J. (2011). *Why some politicians are more dangerous than others.* Polity.

Gilmore, R. W. (2022). *Abolition geography: Essays towards liberation.* Verso.

Ginwright, S. (2016). *Hope and healing in urban education: How urban activists and teachers are reclaiming matters of the heart.* Routledge.

Ginwright, S. (2018, May). The future of healing: Shifting from trauma informed care to healing centered engagement. *Medium.* medium.com/@ginwright/the-future-of-healing-shifting-from-trauma-informed-care-to-healing-centered-engagement-634f557ce69c

Goldberg, H. (2022). Growing brains, nurturing minds—Neuroscience as an educational tool to support students' development and life-long learners. *Brain Science, 12*(12). doi:10.3390/brainsci12121622

Gray, P. (2017). What exactly is play, and why is it such a powerful vehicle for learning? *Topics in Language Disorders, 37*(3), 217–228. doi:10.1097/TLD.0000000000000130

Gray, P., Lancy, D., & Bjorklund, D. (2023). Decline in independent activity as a cause of decline in children's mental well-being: Summary of the evidence. *The Journal of Pediatrics, 260*, 113352. doi: 10.1016/j.jpeds.2023.02.004

Greenberg, M. T. (2023). *Evidence for social and emotional learning in schools.* Learning Policy Institute. doi:10.54300/928.269

Gross, N. (2024). *Brothers in grief: The hidden toll of gun violence on Black boys and their schools.* The University of Chicago Press.

Guarino, K., & Chagnon, E. (2018). *Trauma-sensitive schools training package.* National Center on Safe Supportive Learning Environments. eric.ed.gov/?id=ED595276

Gypen, L., Vanderfaeillie, J., De Maeyer, S., Belenger, L., & Van Holen, F. (2017). Outcomes of children who grew up in foster care: Systematic-review. *Children and Youth Services Review, 76*, 74–83. doi:10.1016/j.childyouth.2017.02.035

Haga, K. (2020). *Healing resistance: A radically different response to harm.* Parallax Press.

Hager, E. (2022, October 13). *Police need warrants to search homes. Child welfare agents almost never get one.* ProPublica. propublica.org/article/child-welfare-search-seizure-without-warrants

Halberstadt, A. G., Cooke, A. N., Garner, P. W., Hughes, S. A., Oertwig, D., & Neupert, S. D. (2020). Racialized emotion recognition accuracy and anger bias of children's faces. *Emotion, 22*(3), 403–417. doi:10.1037/emo0000756

Hall, W. (2018). Psychosocial risk and protective factors for depression among lesbian, gay, bisexual, and queer youth: A systematic review. *Journal of Homosexuality, 65*(3), 263–316. doi:10.1080/00918369.2017.1317467

Hart Research. (2022). *Under siege: The outlook of AFT members.* aft.org/sites/default/files/media/2022/de-14326_aft_member_survey.pdf

Held, V. (2005). *The ethics of care: Personal, political, and global.* Oxford Academic.

Hertel, R., & Johnson, M. M. (2020). How the traumatic experiences of students manifest in school settings. In E. Rossen (Ed.), *Supporting and educating traumatized students: A guide for school-based professionals* (pp. 27–44). Oxford University Press.

High, A. J. (2017). Using restorative practices to teach and uphold dignity in an American school district. *McGill Journal of Education, 52*(2), 525–534. doi:10.7202/1044479ar

Hochul, C., Fabbi, C., Kimball, A., Bohen, I., & Russo, J. (2025). *School mental health report card.* Inseparable. inseparable.us/wp-content/uploads/dlm_uploads/2025/04/Inseparable-2025SchoolMHReportCard-041625-Full.pdf

Houston, D. M. (2025). The year in public opinion on U.S. K–12 education policy. A review of surveys finds Americans want schools to refocus on teaching and learning. *Education Next, 25*(1), 22–31. educationnext.org/the-year-in-public-opinion-on-u-s-k-12-education-policy/

Hunt-Hendrix, L., & Taylor, A. (2024). *Solidarity: The past, present, and future of a world-changing idea.* Penguin Random House.

Institute of Educational Sciences. (2022). *School pulse panel.* ies.ed.gov/schoolsurvey/spp/

Institute to Transform Child Protection. (2025, April 4). *Reimagining mandated reporting.* [Video]. Vimeo. vimeo.com/1072599814

Irwin, V., Wang, K., Cui, J., Zhang, J., & Thompson, A. (2021). *Report on the indicators of school crime and safety: 2020.* Institute of Education Sciences. nces.ed.gov/pubs2021/2021092.pdf

Ishimaru, A. M. (2017). From family engagement to equitable collaboration. *Educational Policy, 33*(2), 1–36. doi:10.1177/0895904817691841

Itzkowitz, M., & Olson, K. (2022). Closing the front door of child protection: Rethinking mandated reporting. *Child Welfare Journal, 100*(2), 77–98. static1.squarespace.com/static/5f925ec584857f3307673b83/t/66c4dc71b70c6b5dc4e94497/1724177521791/Itzkowitz-Closing+the+Front+Door+of+Child+Protection-+Rethinking+Mandated+Reporting-2022-Child+Welfare.pdf

Itzkowitz, M., & Olson, K. (2023). *Resources for Mandated Reporters.* Institute to Transform Child Protection. transformchildprotection.org/resources-for-mandated-reporters/

Jackson, D., Fahmy, C., Vaughn, M., & Testa, A. (2019). Police stops among at-risk youth: Repercussions for mental health. *The Journal of Adolescent Health, 65*(5), 627–632. doi: 10.1016/j.jadohealth.2019.05.027

Jackson, L. (2016). Why should I be grateful? The morality of gratitude in contexts marked by injustice. *Journal of Moral Education, 45*(3), 1–15. doi:10.1080/03057240.2016.1186612

Jacques, C., & Villegas, A. (2018). *Strategies for equitable family engagement.* State Support Network. ed.gov/sites/ed/files/2020/10/equitable_family_engag_508.pdf

Jaffe, S. (2021). *Work won't love you back: How devotion to our jobs keeps us exploited, exhausted, and alone.* Bold Type Books.

James, A., Kristjánsson, K., & Vogler, C. (2020). Seeking the common good in education through a positive conception of social justice. *British Journal of Educational Studies, 69*(1). doi:10.1080/00071005.2020.1724259

Jaycox, L., Langley, A., & Dean, K. (2009). *Support for students exposed to trauma: The SSET program.* RAND Corporation. rand.org/content/dam/rand/pubs/technical_reports/2009/RAND_TR675.pdf

Jazaieri, H. (2017, February 7). *What we still don't know about mindfulness meditation.* Greater Good Science Center. Retrieved from https://greatergood.berkeley.edu/article/item/what_we_still_dont_know_about_mindfulness_meditation

Jennings, P. A. (2015). *Mindfulness for teachers: Simple skills for peace and productivity in the classroom.* W. W. Norton.

JMACForFamilies. (n.d.). *Mandated Supporting.* jmacforfamilies.org/mandated-supporting

Johnson, C. (2018, November 26). *Understanding the cycle of a meltdown.* Oregon Association for the Education of the Young Child. oraeyc.org/single-post/2018/11/26/Understanding-the-Cycle-of-a-Meltdown

Jones, N., Camburn, E., Kelcey, B., & Quintero, E. (2021). *Teachers' time use and affect before and after COVID-19 school closures.* Wheelock Educational Policy Center. wheelockpolicycenter.org/effective-teachers/teacher-time-use-and-affect-during-covid-19/

Julle-Danière E., Whitehouse J., Mielke, A., Vrij, A., Gustafsson, E., Micheletta, J., & Waller, B. M. . (2020). Are there non-verbal signals of guilt? *PLoS One, 15*(4), e0231756. doi:10.1371/journal.pone.0231756

Justice, B. (2023). Schooling as a white good. *History of Education Quarterly, 63*(2), 154–178. doi:10.1017/heq.2023.7

Kaba, M. (2021). *We do this 'til we free us: Abolitionist organizing and transforming justice.* Haymarket Books.

Kaba, M., & Hayes, K. (2021). The sentencing of Larry Nassar was not 'transformative justice.' Here's why. In M. Kaba (Ed.), *We do this 'til we free us: Abolitionist organizing and transforming justice* (pp. 58–67). Haymarket Books.

Katic, B., Alba, L. A., & Johnson, A. H. (2020). A systematic evaluation of restorative justice practices: School violence prevention and response. *Journal of School Violence, 19*(4),1–15. doi:10.1080/15388220.2020.1783670

Kelty, N. E., & Wakabayashi, T. (2020). Family engagement in schools: Parent, educator, and community perspectives. *SAGE Open, 10*(4), 1–13. doi:10.1177/2158244020973024

Kieran, L., & Anderson, C. (2019). Connecting universal design for learning with culturally responsive teaching. *Education and Urban Society, 51*(9), 1202–1216. doi:10.1177/0013124518785012

Kim, H., & Drake, B. (2018). Child maltreatment risk as a function of poverty and race/ethnicity in the USA. *International Journal of Epidemiology, 47*(3), 780–787. doi:10.1093/ije/dyx280

Kim, H., Wildeman, C., Jonson-Reid, M., & Drake, B. (2017). Lifetime prevalence of investigating child maltreatment. *American Journal of Public Health, 107*(2), 274–280. doi:10.2105/AJPH.2016.303545

Kimmerer, R. W. (2015). *Braiding sweetgrass: Indigenous wisdom, scientific knowledge, and the teachings of plants.* Milkweed Editions.

Kirmayer, L. J., Dandeneau, S., Marshall, E., Phillips, M. K., & Williamson, K. J. (2011). Rethinking resilience from Indigenous perspectives. *Canadian Journal of Psychiatry, 56*(2), 84–91. https://journals.sagepub.com/doi/pdf/10.1177/070674371105600203

Kiss, O., Alzuleta, E., Yuksel, D., Pohl, K., Zambotti, M., Muller-Oehring, E. M. , Prouty, D., Durley, I., Pelham III, W. E., McCabe, C. J., Gonzalez, M. R., Brown, S. A., Wade, N. E., Marshall, A. T., Sowell, E. R., Breslin, F. J., LIsdahl, K. M., Dick, A. S., Sheth, C. S., McCandliss, B. D., Guillaume, M., Van Rinsveld, A. M., Dowling, G. J., Tapert, S. F., & Baker, F. C. (2022). The pandemic's toll on young adolescents: Prevention and intervention targets to preserve their mental health. *Journal of Adolescent Health, 70*(3), 387–395. doi: 10.1016/j.jadohealth.2021.11.023

Klein, N. (2024). *Doppelganger: A trip into the mirror world.* Picador Paper.

Kopec, D., & Harte, J. (2020). Design as the missing variable in trauma-informed schools. In E. Rossen (Ed.), *Supporting and educating traumatized students: A guide for school-based professionals* (2nd ed., pp. 343–357). Oxford University Press.

Krase, K. S. (2013). Education personnel as reporters of suspected child maltreatment. *Child & Schools, 35*(3), 147–154. doi:10.1093/cs/cdt008

Krawec, P. (2022). *Becoming kin: An Indigenous call to unforgetting the past and reimagining our future.* Broadleaf Books.

Kurtz, H., Lloyd, S., Harwin, A., Comai, S., & Gong, R. (2024). *Understanding school climate and student well-being: Results of national surveys.* EdWeek Research Center. edweek.org/research-center/leadership/reports/understanding-school-climate-and-student-well-being-results-of-national-surveys

Kuyken, W., Ball, S., Crane, C., Ganguli, P., Jones, B., Montero-Marin, J., Nuthall, E., Raja, A., Taylor, L.,

Tudor, K., Viner, R., Allwood, M., Aukland, L., Dunning, D., Casey, T., Dalrymple, N., De Wilde, K., Farley, E., Harper, J., Hinze, V., Kappelmann, N., Kempnich, M., Lord, L., Medlicott, E., Palmer, L., Petit, A., Philips, A., Pryor-Nitsch, I., Radley, L., Sonley, A., Shackleford, J., Tickell, A., Team, M., Blakemore, S-J., Ukoumunne, O., Greenberg, M., Ford, T., Dalgleish, T., Byford, S., & Williams, J. M. G. (2022, July). Effectiveness of universal school-based mindfulness training compared with normal school provision on teacher mental health and school climate: results of the MYRIAD cluster randomised controlled trial. *Evidence-Based Mental Health*. doi:10.1136/ebmental-2022-300424

Lawson, H. A., Caringi, J. C., Gottfried, R., Bride, B. E., & Hydon, S. P. (2019, September 1). Educators' secondary traumatic stress, children's trauma, and the need for trauma literacy. *Harvard Educational Review, 89*(3), 421–447. doi:10.17763/1943-5045-89.3.421

L. B. v. The City of New York et al., No. 23-CV-8501 (S.D.N.Y. 2025).

Legewie, J., & Fagan, J. (2019). Aggressive policing and the educational performance of minority youth. *American Sociological Review, 82*(2), 220–247. doi.org/10.1177/0003122419826020

Levey, E., Gelaye, B., Bain, P., Rondon, M., Borba, C., Henderson, D., & Williams, M. (2017). A systematic review of randomized control trials of interventions designed to decrease child abuse in high-risk families. *Child Abuse & Neglect, 65*, 48–57. doi.org/10.1016/j.chiabu.2017.01.004

Lewallen, T. C., Hunt, H., Potts-Datema, W., Zaza, S., & Giles, W. (2015). The whole school, whole community, whole child model: A new approach for improving educational attainment and healthy development for students. *Journal of School Health, 85*(11), 729–739. doi:10.1111/josh.12310

Link, B. G., & Phelan, J. (1995). Social conditions as fundamental causes of disease. *Journal of Health and Social Behavior,* 80–94. doi:10.2307/2626958

Liu, J., Ein, N., Gervasio, J., Battaion, M., Reed, M., & Vickers, K. (2020). Comprehensive meta-analysis of resilience interventions. *Clinical Psychology Review, 82*, 101919. doi:10.1016/j.cpr.2020.101919

Lloyd, A., & Borrill, J. (2020). Examining the effectiveness of restorative justice in reducing victims' post-traumatic stress. *Psychological Injury and Law,13*, 77–89. doi:10.1007/s12207-019-09363-9

Lo, C. K.-M., & Cho, Y. W. (2021). Community-based interventions to reduce child maltreatment. *Research on Social Work Practice, 31*(6), 621–633. doi:10.1177/1049731520986968

Lodi, E., Perrella, L., Lepri, G. L., Scarpa, M. L., & Patrizi, P. (2022, December 23). Use of restorative justice and restorative practices at school: A systematic literature review. *International Journal of Environmental Research and Public Health, 19*(1), 96. doi:10.3390/ijerph19010096

López-Castro, T., Saraiya, T., Zumberg-Smith, K., & Dambreville, N. (2019). Association between shame and posttraumatic stress disorder: A meta-analysis. *Journal of Traumatic Stress, 32*(4), 484–495. doi:10.1002/jts.22411

López-Pérez, B., & Pacella, D. (2021). Interpersonal emotion regulation in children: Age, gender, and cross-cultural differences using a serious game. *Emotion, 21*(1), 17–27. doi:10.1037/emo0000690

Lowry, R., Kennedy, K., & Johns, M. M., Harper, C. R., & Wilkins, N. J. (2022). Associations between school absence and school violence by sexual identity. *American Journal of Preventive Medicine, 63*(3), 384–391. doi:10.1016/j.amepre.2022.03.026

MacLeod, J., & Nelson, G. (2000). Programs for the promotion of family wellness and the prevention of child maltreatment: A meta-analytic review. *Child Abuse & Neglect, 24*(9), 1127–1149. doi:10.1016/s0145-2134(00)00178-2

MacPhail, T. [@drtheresamacphail]. (2024, January 7). *Here's something I added to all my syllabi recently.* [Thread]. Threads. threads.net/@drtheresamacphail/post/C10Q900LKXj/?igshid=NTc4MTIwNjQ2YQ%3D%3D

Madea, A. (2018). C3 De-escalation workbook.

Maier, A., Daniel, J., Oakes, J., & Lam, L. (2017). *Community schools as an effective school improvement strategy: A review of the evidence.* Learning Policy Institute. learningpolicyinstitute.org/product/community-schools-effective-school-improvement-report

Malvaso, C., Pilkington, R., Montgomerie, A., Delfabbro, P., & Lynch, J. (2020). A public health approach to preventing child maltreatment: An intelligent information infrastructure to help us know what works. *Child Abuse & Neglect, 106*, 104466. doi:10.1016/j.chiabu.2020.104466

Mangelsdorf, J., Eid, M., & Luhmann, M. (2018). Does growth require suffering? A systematic review and meta-analysis on genuine posttraumatic and postecstatic growth. *Psychological Bulletin, 145*(3), 302–338. doi:10.1037/bul0000173

Marya, R., & Patel, R. (2021). *Inflamed: Deep medicine and the anatomy of injustice.* Farrar, Straus and Giroux.

Mayes, K. A. (2022). *The unteachables: Disability rights and the invention of Black special education.* University of Minnesota Press.

Maynard, B. R., Farina, A., Dell, N. A., & Kelly, M. S. (2019). Effects of trauma-informed approaches in schools: A systematic review. *Campbell Systematic Reviews, 15*(1-2). doi.org/10.1002/cl2.1018

Mayte, M. [@couldbe_mayte]. (2023, November 4). *I don't have allyship fatigue.* [Video]. TikTok. tiktok.com/@couldbe_mayte/video/7297380157487123755

McCartin, J. A. (2016). Bargaining for the common good. *Dissent, 63*(2), 128–135. doi:10.1353/dss.2016.0029

McCarthy, J. E., & Rubinstein, S. A. (2018, October). *National study on union-management partnerships and educator collaboration in US public schools.* Rutgers School of Management and Labor Relations. cdefoundation.org/staging/wp-content/uploads/2018/02/Cornell-Rutgers-Working-Paper-10-13-17.pdf

McDonald. (2013). Labor arbitration decision. 148115-AAA, 2013 BNA LA Supp. 148115.

McKnight, K., Venkateswaran, N., Laird, J., Robles, J., & Shalev, T. (2017). *Mindset shifts and parent teacher home visits.* RTI International. pthvp.org/wp-content/uploads/2022/03/mindset-shifts-and-parent-teacher-home-visits.pdf

McMahon, S., Anderman, E., Astor, R., Espelage, D., Martinez, A., Reddy, L., & Worrell, F. (2022). *Violence against educators and school personnel: Crisis during COVID.* American Psychological Association. apa.org/education-career/k12/violence-educators.pdf

McPherson, K. (2021). Are we free to go? Anti-Black racism and its impact on Black play. *American Journal of Play, 13*(2-3), 356–382. museumofplay.org/app/uploads/2022/01/13-2-Article-12-Free-to-go.pdf

McTavish, J., Kimber, M., Devries, K., Colombini, M., MacGregor, J., Wathen, C., Agarwal, A., & MacMillan, H. (2017). Mandated reporters' experiences with reporting child maltreatment: A meta-synthesis of qualitative studies. *BMJ Open,* 7(10). doi: 10.1136/bmjopen-2016-013942

Meier v. Salem-Keizer School District, A155836,_P.3d_(Or. Ct. App. 2017).

Menesini, E., & Salmivalli, C. (2017). Bullying in schools: The state of knowledge and effective interventions. *Psychology, Health & Medicine, 22*, 240–253. doi.org/10.1080/13548506.2017.1279740

Merkel-Holguin, L., Drury, I., Gibley-Reed, C., Lara, A., Jihad, M., Grint, K., & Marlowe, K. (2022). Structures of oppression in the U.S. child welfare system: Reflections on administrative barriers to equity. *Societies, 12*(26). mdpi.com/2075-4698/12/1/26/pdf

Merrick, M., Ford, D., Ports, K., & Guinn, A. (2018). Prevalence of adverse childhood experiences from the 2011–2014 behavioral risk factor surveillance system in 23 states. *JAMA Pediatrics, 172*(11), 1038–1044. doi:10.1001/jamapediatrics.2018.2537

Merrick, M., Ford, D., Ports, K., Guinn, A., Chen, J., Klevens, J., Metzler, M., Jones, C.M., Simon, T.R., Daniel, V.M., Ottley, P., & Mercy, J. (2019, November 8). Vital signs: Estimated proportion of adult health problems attributable to adverse childhood experiences and implications for prevention - 25 states, 2015–2017. *Morbidity and Mortality Weekly Report, 68*(44), 999–1005. doi:10.15585/mmwr.mm6844e1

Meyers, S., Rowell, K., Wells, M., & Smith, B. C. (2019). Teacher empathy: A model of empathy for teaching of student success. *College Teaching, 67*(3), 160–168. doi:10.1080/87567555.2019.1579699

National Association for Family, School, and Community Engagement. (2022). *Family engagement core competencies: A body of knowledge, skills, and dispositions for family-facing professionals.* nafsce.org/

page/CoreCompetencies

National Child Traumatic Stress Network Schools Committee. (2008, October). *Child trauma toolkit for educators*. National Center for Child Traumatic Stress (NCTSN). nctsn.org/resources/child-trauma-toolkit-educators

National Labor Relations Board. (n.d.). *Concerted activity.* nlrb.gov/about-nlrb/rights-we-protect/the-law/employees/concerted-activity

National Scientific Council on the Developing Child. (2015). *Supportive relationships and active skill-building strengthen the foundations of resilience: Working Paper 13.* Center on the Developing Child, Harvard University. chrome-extension://efaidnbmnnnibpcajpcglclefindmkaj/https://developingchild.harvard.edu/wp-content/uploads/2024/10/The-Science-of-Resilience2.pdf

Newland, B. (2022). *Federal Indian boarding school initiative investigative report.* U.S. Bureau of Indian Affairs. bia.gov/sites/default/files/dup/inline-files/bsi_investigative_report_may_2022_508.pdf

Office of the Surgeon General. (2024). *Parents under pressure: The U.S. Surgeon General's advisory on the mental health and well-being of parents.* U.S. Department of Health and Human Services. hhs.gov/surgeongeneral/priorities/parents/index.html

Ollison, J. (2019). *Improving teacher retention by addressing teachers' compassion fatigue* [Doctoral Dissertation, University of the Pacific]. University of the Pacific Theses and Dissertations. scholarlycommons.pacific.edu/uop_etds/3602

Onyeka-Crawford, A., Patrick, K., & Chaudhry, N. (2017). *Let her learn: Stopping school pushout for girls of color.* National Women's Law Center. nwlc.org/wp-content/uploads/2017/04/final_nwlc_Gates_GirlsofColor.pdf

Osborne-Crowley, L. (2020, April 16). *How shame makes us sick*. Wellcome Collection. wellcomecollection.org/stories/XoR36xIAAPzSyP9D

Pac, J., Collyer, S., Berger, L., O'Brien, K., Parker, E., Pecora, P., Rostad, W., Waldfogel, J., & Wimer, C. (2023). The effects of child poverty reductions on child protective services involvement. *Social Service Review, 97*(1), 43–91. journals.uchicago.edu/doi/epdf/10.1086/723219

Palmer, L., Font, S., Eastman, A. L., Guo, L., & Putnam-Hornstein, E. (2024). What does child protective services investigate as neglect? A population-based study. *Child Maltreatment, 29*(1), 96–105. doi:10.1177/10775595221114144

Palmer, L., Font, S., Rebbe, R., & Putnam-Hornstein, E. (2023). Lifetime rates and types of subsequent child protection system contact following a first report of neglect: An age-stratified analysis. *PLoS One, 18*(4), e0283534. doi:10.1371/journal.pone.0283534

Palusci, V., & Botash, A. (2021). Race and bias in child maltreatment diagnosis and reporting. *Pediatrics, 148*(1), e2020049625. doi:10.1542/peds.2020-049625

Parameswaran, U. D., Molloy, J., & Kuttner, P. (2023). Healing schools: A framework for joining trauma-informed care, restorative justice, and multicultural education for whole school reform. *The Urban Review, 56*, 186–209. doi:10.1007/s11256-023-00666-5

Parent Teacher Home Visits. (2023). *25 years of impact: 25 stories that have shaped a movement to build relational trust between schools and families.* pthvp.org/wp-content/uploads/2023/06/PTHV-Impact-Report-web2.pdf

Partnership for the Future of Learning. (n.d.). *Community schools playbook.* https://communityschools.futureforlearning.org/assets/downloads/community-schools-playbook.pdf

Pascoe, M., Thompson, D., Jenkins, Z., & Ski, C. (2017). Mindfulness mediates the physiological markers of stress: Systematic review and meta-analysis. *Journal of Psychiatric Research, 95*(2017), 156–178. doi.org/10.1016/j.jpsychires.2017.08.004

Peltier, M. R., Edwards, P. R., Sweeney, J., Reichmuth, H. L., White, K. L., Rice, D. R., & Castle, A. (2025). Exploring how educators perceive enacting asset-based family engagement. *Social Sciences, 14*(4),

191. doi:10.3390/socsci14040191

People v. Davis, E034765 (Cal. Ct. App. 2005).

Perry, B. (2020, April 2). *5. Understanding regulation: Neurosequential network stress & trauma series* [Video]. Info NMN. youtube.com/watch?v=L3qlYGwmHYY

Petrone, R., & Rogers Stanton, C. (2021, May). From producing to reducing trauma: A call for "trauma-informed" researchers to interrogate how schools harm students. *Education Researcher, 50*(8). doi:https://doi.org/10.3102/0013189X211014850

Pfeffer, J. (2018). *Dying for a paycheck: How modern management harms employee health and company performance—and what we can do about it.* Harper Collins.

Phifer, L. W. (2020). Students exposed to domestic violence. In E. Rossen (Ed.), *Supporting and educating traumatized students: A guide for school-based professionals* (pp. 195–207). Oxford University Press.

The Philadelphia Public School Notebook. (2020, September 4). *Here we're not outcasts* [Video]. Chalkbeat. youtube.com/watch?v=j408aFc62KU

Pickens, I. (2020). A trauma-informed and culturally responsive approach in the classroom. In E. Rossen (Ed.), *Supporting and educating traumatized students: A guide for school-based professionals* (pp. 45–58). Oxford University Press.

Pietrantoni, Z., Chitiyo, J., Chitiyo, A., Peña, J., & Fernandez, K. (2023, June). Perceived preparedness of school practitioners to identify and report child maltreatment. *Social Development Issues, 45*(3). doi:10.3998/sdi.4487

Posamentier, J., Seibel, K., & DyTang, N. (2022). Preventing youth suicide: A review of school-based practices and how social–emotional learning fits into comprehensive efforts. *Trauma, Violence & Abuse, 24*(2). doi:10.1177/15248380211039475

Prax, C. (2015). *Helping children thrive: Child health survey report.* AFT. aft.org/sites/default/files/media/2015/helpingchildrenthrive2015.pdf

Prax, C. (2025). *Nobody wins: Educators' perspectives on mandatory reporting.* AFT, UC Irvine. bit.ly/NobodyWins-ToMandatedSupport

Prax, C., & Acosta Price, O. (2025). *Mandated supporters in education: Wrap around the family.* AFT and The Center for Health and Health Care in Schools. aft.org/sites/default/files/media/documents/2025/aft-chhcs2025_mandated_supporters-wrap_around_the_family.pdf

Prax, C., & O'Connor, B. (2018). *School personnel can help students heal from trauma.* AFT and Futures Without Violence. aft.org/school-personnel-can-help-students-heal-trauma

Prax, C., Paxson, A., Mandle, J., & Marcy, C. (2025, March). *Mandated supporters in education: Build healing relationships with students and families.* AFT and Healthy Schools Campaign. aft.org/sites/default/files/media/documents/2025/aft-hsc2025_mandated_supporters_build_healing_relationships.pdf

Proeschold-Bell, R. J., Sohail, M. M., Huynh, H., Baghdady, A., Vann, V., Amanya, C., Al-Khalaf, M., & Whetten, K. (2021). *Teacher wellbeing: Findings from a scoping literature review and case studies in Cambodia, Kenya, and Qatar.* World Innovation Summit for Education. wise-qatar.org/app/uploads/2021/11/2021wise-rr4-report-web-version.pdf

Pryce, J. (2024). *Broken: Transforming child protective services—notes of a former caseworker.* Amistad.

Ramstetter, C., & Murray, R. (2017). Time to play: Recognizing the benefits of recess. *American Educator, 41*(1), 17–23, 43. aft.org/ae/spring2017

Raz, M. (2020). *Abusive policies: How the American child welfare system lost its way.* The University of North Carolina Press.

REX TV by YouthREX. (2021, February 19). *From trauma-informed care to healing-centered engagement: A #YouthWork teach-in with Dr. Shawn Ginwright* [Video]. YouTube. youtube.com/watch?v=NxTSIlWUeg8

Richards, T., & Fromknecht. (2024). Measuring due process and fairness in the child welfare court system.

Juvenile and Family Court Journal, 75, 27–43. doi:10.1111/jfcj.12258

Ritch, J. (Host). (2014). Extraenvironmentalist #51 [Audio Podcast]. In *Culture of Dying*. Orphan Wisdom. soundcloud.com/orphan-wisdom/stephen-jenkinson-culture-of-dying

Roberts, D. (2022). *Torn apart: How the child welfare system destroys Black families—and how abolition can build a safer world.* Basic Books.

Roe v. Hesperia Unified School District, E075092 (Cali. Ct. App. 2022).

Rogers, C. (1957). The necessary and sufficient conditions of therapeutic personality change. *Journal of Consulting Psychology, 21*(2), 95–103. doi:10.1037/h0045357

Rogers, R., & Sears, S. (2015). Emotional Freedom Techniques (EFT) for stress in students: A randomized controlled dismantling study. *Energy Psychology*, 26–32. focusedhealthyfamily.com/wp-content/uploads/2016/07/College-Student-EFT-Study.pdf

Rohde-Collins, D. (2020). Students exposed to community violence. In E. Rossen (Ed.), *Supporting and educating traumatized students: A guide for school-based professionals* (pp. 126–163). Oxford University Press.

Ross, E. M. (2023, March 21). *The case for strong family and community engagement in schools*. Harvard Graduate School of Education. gse.harvard.edu/ideas/usable-knowledge/23/03/case-strong-family-and-community-engagement-schools

Rudolph, J., & Zimmer-Gembeck, M. J. (2018). Reviewing the focus: A summary and critique of child-focused sexual abuse prevention. *Trauma, Violence, & Abuse, 19*(5), 543–554. doi:10.1177/1524838016675478

Russell, J. R., Kerwin, C., & Halverson, J. L. (2018). Is child protective services effective? *Children and Youth Services Review, 84*, 185–192. doi:10.1016/j.childyouth.2017.11.028

Ruttenberg, D. (2022). *On repentance and repair: Making amends in an unapologetic world.* Beacon Press.

Sabol, T. J., Kessler, C. L., Rogers, L. O., Petitclerc, A., Silver, J., Briggs-Gowan, M., & Wakschlag, L. S. (2022). A window into racial and socioeconomic status disparities in preschool disciplinary action using developmental methodology. *Annals of the New York Academy of Sciences, 1508*(1), 123–136. doi:10.1111/nyas.14687

Salter, M., & Hall, H. (2020). Reducing shame, promoting dignity: A model for the primary prevention of complex post-traumatic stress disorder. *Trauma, Violence & Abuse, 23*(3), 1–14. doi:10.1177/1524838020979667

Sanchis-Sanchis, A., Grau, M. D., Moliner, A.-R., & Morales-Murillo, C. P. (2020). Effects of age and gender in emotion regulation of children and adolescents. *Frontiers in Psychology, 11*, 946. doi:10.3389/fpsyg.2020.00946

Sanders, J., Joseph-McCatty, A., Massey, M., Swiatek, E., Csiernik, B., & Igor, E. (2023). Exposure to adversity and trauma among students who experience school discipline: A scoping review. *Review of Educational Research, 94*(5), 699–724. doi:10.3102/00346543231203674

Sankaran, V., Church, C., & Mitchell, M. (2019). A cure worse than the disease? The impact of removal on children and their families. *Marquette Law Review, 102*(4), 1163–94. https://repository.law.umich.edu/cgi/viewcontent.cgi?article=3055&context=articles

Schibalski, J., Muller, M., Ajdacic-Gross, V., Vetter, S., Rodgers, S., Oexle, N., Corrigan, P., Rossler, W., & Rusch, N. (2017). Trauma-related stress, shame and avoidant coping reactions among members of the general population with elevated symptoms. *Comprehensive Psychiatry, 74*(April 2017), 224–230. doi:10.1016/j.comppsych.2017.02.001

Schmidt, C. N., Stretten, M., & Briscoe, H. (2021). Widespread surveillance by the child protection system: Lasting effects on families. *American Journal of Public Health, 111*(12), e1–e2. doi: 10.2105/AJPH.2021.306530

Schonfeld, D., & Quackenbush, M. (2021). *The grieving student: A guide for schools.* Paul H. Brookes

Publishing Co, Inc.

Sciacca, A. (2023, October 11). You have the right to refuse CPS entry: Texas launches Miranda-style warnings to parents under investigation for child maltreatment. *The Imprint*. imprintnews.org/top-stories/you-have-the-right-to-refuse-cps-entry-texas-launches-miranda-style-warnings-to-parents-under-investigation-for-child-maltreatment/245334

Scotland-Coogan, D., & Davis, E. (2016). Relaxation techniques for trauma. *Journal of Evidence-Informed Social Work, 13*(5), 434–441. doi:10.1080/23761407.2016.1166845

Semerci, R., Öztürk, G., Akgün Kostak, M., Elmas, S., İhsan Danacı, A., & Musbeg, S. (2020). The effect of progressive muscle relaxation exercises on compassion satisfaction, burnout, and compassion fatigue of nurse managers. *Perspectives in Psychiatric Care, 57*(3), 1250–1256. doi:10.1111/ppc.12681

Shalaby, C. (2017). *Troublemakers: Lessons in freedom from young children at school.* The New Press.

Shapiro, D. L. (2021). Reconciliation systems design: A systematic approach to collective healing in post-conflict societies. *Harvard Negotiation Law Review, 26*(193), 194–264. journals.law.harvard.edu/hnlr/wp-content/uploads/sites/91/26-HNLR-193-Shapiro.pdf

Sheldon, S. B., & Jung, S. B. (2018). *Student outcomes and parent teacher home visits.* Johns Hopkins School of Education. pthvp.org/wp-content/uploads/2022/03/student-outcomes-and-parent-teacher-home-visits.pdf

Shew, A. (2023). *Against technoableism: Rethinking who needs improvement.* W. W. Norton & Company.

Shi, C., Ren, Z., Zhao, C., & Chan, S. H.-W. (2021). Shame, guilt, and posttraumatic stress symptoms: A three-level meta-analysis. *Journal of Anxiety Disorders, 82*, 102443. doi:10.1016/j.janxdis.2021.102443

Shlasko, D. (2015). Using the five faces of oppression to teach about interlocking systems of oppression. *Equity & Excellence in Education, 48*(3), 349–360. doi:10.1080/10665684.2015.1057061

Siegel, A., Esqueda, M. C., Berkowitz, R., Sullivan, K., Astor, R. A., & Benbenishty, R. (2018). Welcoming parents to their child's school: Practices supporting students with diverse needs and backgrounds. *Education and Urban Society, 51*(6), 001312451774768. doi:10.1177/0013124517747682

Simmons-Duffin, S. (2018, May 23). *To teach kids to handle tough emotions, some schools take time out for group therapy.* NPR. npr.org/sections/health-shots/2018/05/23/613465023/for-troubled-kids-some-schools-take-time-out-for-group-therapy

Skulina, T. R. (2010). Labor arbitration decision. Orange County Public Schools, 09 (0521) - 57084-3, 127 BNA LA 737.

Slack, K., & Berger, L. (2020). Who is and is not served by child protective systems? Implications for a prevention infrastructure to reduce child maltreatment. The ANNALS of the American Academy of Political and Social Science, 692(1), 182–202. doi:10.1177/0002716220980691

Smith, C. (2022). *How the word is passed: A reckoning with the history of slavery across America.* Little, Brown and Company.

Smith Lee, J. R., & Robinson, M. A. (2019). "That's my number one fear in life. It's the police.": Examining young Black men's exposures to trauma and loss resulting from police violence and police killings. *Journal of Black Psychology, 45*(3), 143–184. doi:10.1177/0095798419865152

Sokolower, J. (2018). Teaching Haniyah. In D. Watson, J. Hagopian, & W. Au (Eds.), *Teaching for Black lives* (pp. 260–263). Rethinking Schools.

Sonsteng-Person, M., & Loomis, A. M. (2021). The role of trauma-informed training in helping Los Angeles teachers manage the effects of student exposure to violence and trauma. *Journal of Child and Adolescent Trauma, 14*(2), 189–199. doi:10.1007/s40653-021-00340-6

Souers, K., & Hall, P. (2016). *Fostering resilient learners: Strategies for creating a trauma-sensitive classroom.* ASCD.

Stamm, H. E., Higson-Smith, C., Hudnall, A. C., Piland, N. F., & Hudnall Stamm, B. (2012). *Professional*

Quality of Worklife (ProQOL 5). The Center for Victims of Torture. proqol.org/

Stand Together. (2023, March 29). *How to raise fearless children* [Video]. YouTube. youtube.com/watch?v=BFQ3QD9JklM

Statista. (2020, June). *Reported number of slaves owned by U.S. presidents who served from 1789 to 1877*. statista.com/statistics/1121963/slaves-owned-by-us-presidents/

Stearns, P. N., & Stearns, C. (2016). American schools and the uses of shame: An ambiguous history. *History of Education, 46*(1), 58–75. doi:10.1080/0046760x.2016.1185671

Stefanski, A., Valli, L., & Jacobson, R. (2016). Beyond involvement and engagment: The role of the family in school-community partnerships. *School Community Journal, 26*(2), 135–160. files.eric.ed.gov/fulltext/EJ1124001.pdf

Steiner, E. D., Doan, S., Woo, A., Gittens, A. D., Lawrence, R. A., Berdie, L., Wolfe, R., Greer, L., & Schwartz, H. L. (2022). *Restoring teacher and principal well-being is an essential step for rebuilding schools*. RAND Corporation. rand.org/content/dam/rand/pubs/research_reports/RRA1100/RRA1108-4/RAND_RRA1108-4.pdf

Steiner, E. D., & Woo, A. (2021). *Job-related stress threatens the teacher supply: Findings from the 2021 State of the U.S. Teacher Survey*. RAND Corporation. rand.org/pubs/research_reports/RRA1108-1.html

Stoltzfus, E. (2024). *Child welfare: Purposes, federal programs, and funding*. Congressional Research Service. crsreports.congress.gov/product/pdf/IF/IF10590

Substance Abuse and Mental Health Services Administration. (2014). *Concept of trauma and guidance for a trauma-informed approach*. U.S. Department of Health and Human Services. store.samhsa.gov/product/SAMHSA-s-Concept-of-Trauma-and-Guidance-for-a-Trauma-Informed-Approach/SMA14-4884.html

Sullivan, M. (2020). Research and best practices to support students with incarcerated parents. In E. Rossen (Ed.), *Supporting and educating traumatized students: A guide for school-based professionals* (pp. 165–179). Oxford University Press.

Sweeney, B., & Caringi, J. (2020). Addressing secondary traumatic stress in trauma-informed schools. In E. Rossen (Ed.)., *Supporting and educating traumatized students* (pp. 313–324). Oxford University Press.

Táíwò, O. (2022). *Elite capture: How the powerful took over identity politics (and everything else)*. Haymarket Books.

Táíwò, O. O., Fehrenbacher, A. E., & Cooke, A. (2021). Material insecurity, racial capitalism, and public health. *Hastings Center Report, 51*(6), 17–22. doi:10.1002/hast.1293

Tangney, J. (2008, February 9). *Shame and guilt: The good, the bad, and the ugly*. [Video]. YouTube. youtube.com/watch?v=febgutDYP7w

Thiesen-Womersley, G. (2021). *Trauma and resilience among displaced populations: A sociocultural exploration*. Springer. doi:10.1007/978-3-030-67712-1

Thobani, S. (2024). What do apologies apologize for? Rearrangements of state violence. *State Crime Journal, 12*(2), 187–205. doi: 10.13169/statecrime.12.2.0187

Thomas, L. (2017). Classroom management techniques. *Managing Behaviors in School Communities*. AFT.

Tippett, K. (Host). (2015). Bessel van der Kolk - Restoring the body: Yoga, EMDR, and treating trauma [Audio Podcast]. In *On Being*. soundcloud.com/onbeing/bessel-van-der-kolk-restoring-the-body-yoga-emdr-and-treating-trauma

Trent, M., Dooley, D. G., & Douge, J. (2019, August). The Impact of racism on child and adolescent health. *Pediatrics 144*(2), 2019–1765. doi:10.1542/peds.2019-1765

Trey. (2024, February 25). *Rest is not resistance, and that is OK: Cancer, grief, & Audre Lorde*. What's One More Pothos. whatsonemorepothos.com/post/rest-is-not-resistance-and-that-is-ok-on-cancer-grief-audre-lorde

Trey. (2025, February 9). Play is political: On white supremacy's denial of Blackness. *What's One More*

Pothos. whatsonemorepothos.com/post/play-is-political-on-white-supremacy-s-denial-of-black-play

Trivedi, S. (2019). The harm of child removal. *N.Y.U. Review of Law & Social Change, 43*, 523–580. scholarworks.law.ubalt.edu/cgi/viewcontent.cgi?article=2087&context=all_fac

Trivedi, S. (2025, February 19). Prof. Shanta Trivedi on a bill that 'puts marginalized families on an equal footing with their more privileged counterparts.' *NCCPR Child Welfare Blog*. nccprblog.org/2025/02/prof-shanta-trivedi-on-bill-that-puts.html

Ungar, M. (2013). Resilience, trauma, context, and culture. *Trauma, Violence, & Abuse, 14*(3), 255–266. doi:10.1177/1524838013487805

Valdez, C. (2023). Trauma, anger, grief & healing: A portrait of an elementary school. *Journal of Trauma Studies in Education, 2*(3), 73–87. doi:10.32674/jtse.v2i3.5772

van der Put, C., Assink, M., Gubbels, J., & van Solinge, N. (2018). Identifying effective components of child maltreatment interventions: A meta-analysis. *Clinical Child and Family Psychology Review, 21*, 171–202. doi:10.1007/s10567-017-0250-5

Venet, A. S. (2019). Role-clarity and boundaries for trauma-informed teachers. *Educational Considerations, 44*(2). doi:10.4148/0146-9282.2175

Venet, A. S. (2021). *Equity-centered trauma-informed education*. W. W. Norton & Company.

Venkateswaran, N., Laird, J., Robles, J., & Jeffries, J. (2018). *Parent teacher home visits implementation study*. RTI International. pthvp.org/wp-content/uploads/2022/03/parent-teacher-home-visits-implementation-study.pdf

Vickers, E. (2019). Unexpected trauma in oral interviewing. *46*(1). *Oral History in Review*. researchonline.ljmu.ac.uk/id/eprint/9863/8/Vickers_Unexpected%20Trauma%20in%20Oral%20Interviewing_final%20for%20production.pdf

Vitucci, R., & Brown, M. (2019). Cultivating teacher leaders: A union-led effort connects classroom practice to education policy. *American Educator*, 4–11. aft.org/ae/spring2019/vitucci_brown

Vloet, T. D., Vloet, A., Bürger, A., & Romanos, M. (2017). Post-traumatic growth in children and adolescents. *Journal of Traumatic Stress Disorders and Treatment, 6*(4). doi:10.4172/2324-8947.1000182

Vulcan, M. (2021). The "muscles of the psyche:" From body literacy to motional literacy. *Frontiers in Psychology, 11*. doi:10.3389/fpsyg.2020.548964

Wachs, S., Bilz, L., Niproschke, S., & Schubarth, W. (2018). Bullying intervention in schools: A multilevel analysis of teachers' success in handling bullying from the students' perspective. *The Journal of Early Adolescence, 39*(5), 1–27. doi: 10.1177/0272431618780423

Walker, L., Tarutani, C., & Furman, B. (2017). The power of restorative apologies (real and imagined) for victims and offenders. *Temida, 20*(3), 435–458. doi:10.2298/TEM1703435W

Wallis, C. (2020, June 12). Why racism, not race, is a risk factor for dying of COVID-19. *Scientific American*. scientificamerican.com/article/why-racism-not-race-is-a-risk-factor-for-dying-of-covid-191/

Walsh, K., Eggins, E., Hine, L., Mathews, B., Kenny, M., Howard, S., Ayling, N., Dallaston, E., Pink, E., & Vagenas, D. (2022). Child protection training for professionals to improve reporting of child abuse and neglect. *Cochrane Database of Systematic Reviews 7*(7), CD011775. doi:10.1002/14651858.CD011775.pub2

Warren, C. A. (2014). Towards a pedagogy for the application of empathy in culturally diverse classrooms. *The Urban Review, 46*, 395–419. doi:10.1007/s11256-013-0262-5

Washington State Legislature. (2024). *Legal defense of a public employee*. app.leg.wa.gov/RCW/default.aspx?cite=26.44.032

Watson, D., Hagopian, J., & Au, W. (Eds.), (2018). *Teaching for Black lives*. Rethinking Schools.

Watson, M., & Ecken, L. (2003). *Learning to trust: Transforming difficult elementary classrooms through developmental discipline*. Jossey-Bass.

Weegar, K. (2019). *Evaluating a child maltreatment training program for elementary school teachers.* University of Ottawa. ruor.uottawa.ca/server/api/core/bitstreams/13bebc3a-9e6b-4241-af6a-4327254d58ae/content

Wenger, E., & Kühn, S. (2021). Neuroplasticity. In T. Strobach, & J. Karbach (Eds.)., *Cognitive Training: An overview of features and applications* (pp. 69–83). Springer. pure.mpg.de/rest/items/item_3190209/component/file_3527168/content

West, N. (Ed.). (2021). *We too: Essays on sex work and survival.* Feminist Press.

Whitbeck, L. B., Adams, G. W., Hoyt, D. R., & Chen, X. (2004). Conceptualizing and measuring historical trauma among American Indian people. *American Journal of Community Psychology, 33*(3-4), 119–130. doi:10.1023/b:ajcp.0000027000.77357.31

Whole Child Model. (2024). *Strong start in a secondary setting.* wholechildmodel.org/secondary-strong-start

Will, M. (2021, September 14). Teachers are not OK, even though we need them to be. *Education Week.* edweek.org/teaching-learning/teachers-are-not-ok-even-though-we-need-them-to-be/2021/09

William, R. F. (2009). Labor arbitration decision. Clatsop County, 126 BNA LA 620.

Wilson, K., Hansen, D., & Li, M. (2011). The traumatic stress response in child maltreatment and resultant neuropsychological effects. *Aggression and Violent Behavior, 16*(2), 87–97. doi:10.1016/j.avb.2010.12.007

Wolmer, L., Hamiel, D., Margalit, N., Versano-Eisman, T., Findler, Y., Laor, N., & Slone, M. (2016). Enhancing children's resilience in schools to confront trauma: The impact on teachers. *Israel Journal of Psychiatry and Related Science, 53*(2), 25–32. researchgate.net/profile/Leo-Wolmer/publication/312129293_Enhancing_Children's_Resilience_in_Schools_to_Confront_Trauma_The_Impact_on_Teachers/links/58b527e945851503bea07f67/Enhancing-Childrens-Resilience-in-Schools-to-Confront-Trauma-The-Impa

Wolmer, L., Laor, N., Dedeoglu, C., Siev, J., & Yazgan, Y. (2005). Teacher-mediated intervention after disaster: A controlled three-year follow-up of children's functioning. *Journal of Child Psychology and Psychiatry, 46*(11), 1161–1168. doi:10.1111/j.1469-7610.2005.00416.x

Wong, Y. J., Cho, N., & Pandelios, A. L. (2024). Feeling good versus doing good: Reclaiming a moral vision for the psychology of gratitude. *International Journal of Applied Positive Psychology, 9*, 1273–1291. doi:10.1007/s41042-024-00157-2

Woo, H., LeTendre, G., Byun, S.-y., & Schussler, D. (2022). Teacher leadership—collective actions, decision-making and well-being. *International Journal of Teacher Leadership, 11*(1), 29–49. files.eric.ed.gov/fulltext/EJ1342978.pdf

Woodnick, G., & Ranney, I. (2022). *A position of trust II: Teachers facing prosecution for failure to report child abuse.* Woodnick Law PLLC. woodnicklaw.com/a-position-of-trust-ii-teachers-facing-prosecution-for-failure-to-report-child-abuse/

Wortley, R., Leclerc, B., Reynald, D. M., & Smallbone, S. (2019). What deters child sex offenders? A comparison between completed and non completed offenses. *Journal of Interpersonal Violence, 34*(20), 4303–4327. doi:10.1177/0886260519869235

Wright, T. (2017). Supporting students who have experienced trauma. *NAMTA Journal, 42*(2), 141–152. files.eric.ed.gov/fulltext/EJ1144506.pdf

Xiaoli, W., Kaminga, A. C., Wenjie, D., Jing, D., Zhipeng, W., Xiongfeng, P., & Aizhong, L. (2019). The prevalence of moderate-to-high posttraumatic growth: A systematic review and meta-analysis. *Journal of Affective Disorders, 243*, 408–415. doi:10.1016/jad.2018.09.023

Yu, X., Sun, C., Sun, B., Yuan, X., Ding, F., & Zhang, M. (2022). The cost of caring: Compassion fatigue is a special form of teacher burnout. *Sustainability, 14*(10), 6071. doi.org/10.3390/su14106071

Yule, K., Houston, J., & Grych, J. (2019). Resilience in children exposed to violence: A meta-analysis of protective factors across ecological contexts. *Clinical Child & Family Psychology Review, 22*, 406-431.

doi: 10.1007/s10567-019-00293-1

Yogman, M., Garner, A., Hutchinson, J., Hirsh-Pasek, K., & Golinkoff, R. M. (2018). The power of play: A pediatric role in enhancing development in young children. *Pediatrics, 142*(3), e20182058. par.nsf.gov/servlets/purl/10119315

Zeng, S., Corr, C. P., O'Grady, C., & Guan, Y. (2019). Adverse childhood experiences and preschool suspension expulsion: A population study. *Child Abuse & Neglect, 97*, 104149. doi:10.1016/j.chiabu.2019.104149

Zimmer-Gembeck, M. J., & Skinner, E. A. (2016). The development of coping: Implications for psychopathology and resilience. In D. Cicchetti, & D. J. Cohen (Eds.), *Developmental psychopathology, volume four, risk, resilience, and intervention.* John Wiley & Sons. doi:10.1002/9781119125556.devpsy410

Zoodsma, M., & Schaafsma, J. (2022). Examining the 'age of apology': Insights from the political apology database. *Journal of Peace Research, 59*(3), 436–448. doi:10.1177/0022343321102469